2151 Old Brick Road
Glen Allen, Va 23060

Negotiating the Holistic Turn

Negotiating the Holistic Turn

*The Domestication
of Alternative Medicine*

JUDITH FADLON

State University of New York Press

Published by
State University of New York Press, Albany

© 2005 State University of New York

All rights reserved

Printed in the United States of America

No part of this book may be used or reproduced in any manner whatsoever without written permission. No part of this book may be stored in a retrieval system or transmitted in any form or by any means including electronic, electrostatic, magnetic tape, mechanical, photocopying, recording, or otherwise without the prior permission in writing of the publisher.

For information, address State University of New York Press,
90 State Street, Suite 700, Albany, NY 12207

Production by Kelli Williams
Marketing by Michael Campochiaro

Library of Congress Cataloging-in-Publication Data

Fadlon, Judith, 1955–
    Negotiating the holistic turn : the domestication of alternative medicine / Judith Fadlon.
    p. cm.
    Includes bibliographical references and index.
    ISBN 0-7914-6315-X (alk. paper) — ISBN 0-7914-6316-8 (pbk. : alk. paper)
    1. Alternative medicine—Israel.   2. Holistic medicine—Israel.
I. Title.
R733.F344 2005
615.5'095694—dc22
                                                                  2004042990

10 9 8 7 6 5 4 3 2 1

*This book is for
Gedi*

Contents

Acknowledgments	ix
Introduction	1
Biomedical Culture Revisited	2
Outline of the Book	6
Chapter 1. Conceptualizing NCM	9
Approaches in the History of NCM Research	9
Domestication: Making Sense of Medicine	16
Acculturation and Assimilation	19
Domestication and the Flow of Culture	23
Chapter 2. Setting the Scene: NCM in Israel	25
The Legal Status of NCM in Israel	27
NCM Institutions in Israel	34
Methodological Considerations	36
Chapter 3. Negotiation: The NCM Clinic	39
The Clinic and Its Boundaries	40
How the Clinic Worked	43
The Staff	47
Case Presentations	51
Chapter 4. The Patients: Group Profile and Patterns of Use	63
Cultural Outlook and the Use of NCM	64
Sociodemographic Characteristics and Health Problems	68
Patients' Attitudes toward Biomedicine	68
Cultural Outlook and Practices	72
The Convergence of Statistics and Ethnography	75

Chapter 5. Dissemination: The Popular Discourse of NCM — 79
Interprofessional Discourse in the Public Arena — 80
The Narrative Formula of Dissemination — 83
Magic Moments — 84
Deus ex Machina—Bio Medicine as the Organizing Principle — 90
Conventional Medicine Fights Back — 91
Horror Stories — 92

Chapter 6. Institutionalization: The NCM College — 97
Introductory Lecture for Potential Students — 100
The Yearbook — 103
The Oriental Medicine Curriculum — 106
The College Bulletin — 111

Chapter 7. Conclusion: Familiarizing the Exotic — 117
Domestication: Clinic, College, Media, and Patients — 119
Local Findings—Global Implications? — 126
Why Domestication? The Interplay between Biomedical Hegemony and Consumerist Demand — 127
The "Other" Appropriated and the "Other" Rejected — 130
NCM and the Postmodern Body — 131

Appendix: NCM Modalities Available at the Clinic — 137
Notes — 143
References — 145
Index — 155

Acknowledgments

I would like to acknowledge a number of individuals who have contributed to my thinking and to this book in particular

I am indebted to Professor Haim Hazan for his intellectual contribution to my work and especially for his kindness, enthusiasm, and encouragement as I progressed from one stage to the next. I would like to thank Professor Yehouda Shenhav for his support and for generously allowing me time to write, and Professor Noah Lewin-Epstein for his contribution at the outset of this project. I also thank Professor Rivka Carmi for her commitment to research and her agenda to support women scholars. My research on alternative medicine has allowed me the privilege of working through my ideas with members of various disciplines. In this capacity, I thank my father, Dr. Gerald Shapiro, for deconstructing boundaries between disciplines, and Professor Shmuel Eidelman for his thoughtful remarks on the reconstruction of those boundaries. Professor Shimon Glick, Professor Micky Weingarten, Professor Carmi Margolis, Dr. Shai Pintov, and Dr. Menachem Oberbaum were exceedingly generous in sharing knowledge, experience, and opinions. Even though we did not always agree, our challenging conversations are undoubtedly reflected in my work.

Ayal Hassidim, who will one day be a healer, has my gratitude for his editorial assistance, and I thank Ilan Roziner for his statistical advice and his rare ability to help me combine ethnography and statistics.

I owe special appreciation to the director, staff, and patients of the clinic where I conducted my fieldwork. I am unable to thank them in name in order to protect the anonymity of the clinic. Thank you.

Beyond the intellectual contribution I have gratefully received in this endeavor, I am indebted to my family for the love, support and indeed, at times, tolerance they have shown. I am obliged to my mother, Sybil, for insisting there is a world outside my study. I thank my partner, Gedi, and my children Thor and Shiri for showing me that world.

My friend, Mercia Hazan, has my gratitude for the invaluable sense of humor and perspective that she brings to our friendship.

An earlier discussion of domestication appeared in Fadlon J. 2004. "Meridians, chakras and psycho-neuro-immunology: The dematerializing body and the domestication of alternative medicine," *Body and Society* 10, 4. Sage Publications.

I would like to thank Laura Ackerman of Hauser Printing Press for her help in designing the emblem on the cover of this book.

Introduction

In recent years, complementary and alternative medicine (often referred to as CAM in the literature) has grown tremendously in both popularity and economic importance. It is now recognized that about one third of the population of industrialized countries has had some experience with CAM. The new medical industry has generated its own field of adherents, practitioners, opponents, lobbyists, counterlobbyists, and regulations. Originally, CAM was regarded as antiestablishment, and the struggle between CAM practitioners and medical doctors has filled volumes of medical, legal, and popular scholarship. In recent years, however, the view of CAM as antiestablishment has changed. It is not the purpose of this book to address the validity of CAM, but rather to focus on social and cultural discourse and the many ways in which CAM is acquiring situated meanings within institutional and social contexts.

Terminology, in the case of CAM, is a charged issue—omnipresent in research on the subject as well as in everyday use. Choice of terminology when discussing the 'other' is highly political, never innocent, and reflects the aspirations of proponents and opponents alike. The problem of selecting the right way to talk about CAM is in fact the same as the problem of how to conceptualize it. In general, terminology used to describe therapeutic methods that do not rest on a Western, scientific rationale has reflected the hegemonic status of biomedical culture. To study the emergence of complementary and alternative medicine is therefore also to study a discourse of social distinction and signification.

In contemporary discourse, the most common terms used to refer to nonconventional medicine are also the most contrasting: "complementary" and "alternative." Practitioners seeking to join up with conventional medicine, or representatives of biomedicine seeking to co-opt and control nonconventional medicine, often use the term "complementary." The term "alternative" is more radical in that it carries the implication of one element replacing another and the concept that nonconventional therapies could, in fact, take the place of conventional medicine in many cases and perhaps compensate for its shortcomings.

To avoid the normative bias of either complementary or alternative, I have chosen to use the term "nonconventional medicine" (NCM for short) as a neutral meeting ground. I use this term whenever referring to therapies that do not draw their theoretical justification from the tradition of modern, Western science. I am well aware that the dichotomy "conventional" versus "nonconventional" is itself weighted with ideology; however, I think it would be naive to assume that a mainstream, conventional form of therapeutic action does not exist within Western society.

This study concerns itself with the dissemination, practice, teaching, and consumption of nonconventional modalities of health treatment in urban Israel. I intend to demonstrate how staff meetings of an NCM clinic are conducted in biomedical terms, how the teaching of NCM is fused with biomedical terminology, how the borders of conventional as well as nonconventional medicine are negotiated in the press, and how NCM consumers don't really seem to differentiate. The key analytical concept suggested here is that of domestication. Domestication, a process in which the foreign is rendered familiar and palatable to local tastes, can explain both the growing popularity of NCM modalities as well as the facility with which individuals move between conventional medicine and NCM modalities, and among the various NCM modalities. Although the focus of this study is urban Israel, I will argue that domestication is a major force behind consumption of medical treatments in a number of settings in Western industrialized countries as well as in low development societies. Despite very different settings, regulatory practices, and the history of contact between systems that are particular to each setting (see, e.g., Baer, 2001; Bishaw, 1991; Bodeker, 2001; Mills, 2001; Saks, 1994), many studies indicate the existence of a uniform process, one that "makes sense of medicine" for consumers. I argue that this process is domestication. Moreover, this study will suggest that domestication illustrates a dynamic process as opposed to other epistemological approaches that have described the static relationship between dominant and imported medical systems.

Biomedical Culture Revisited

Despite postmodern declarations regarding the presumed death of grand (and hence hegemonic) narratives, one such "grand narrative" is alive and well in medicine. This global discourse of Western medicine is commonly referred to as "biomedical culture" by sociologists and has provided an instance of expansion of ideas and practices from the center to the periphery. It is important to understand the 'doxa,' the accepted ideology and practice of biomedical culture, in order to better analyze the heterodoxa (NCM). Biomedical culture encompasses the current practice and ideology of conventional medicine that has historically emerged from modern Western biology (Lock and Gordon, 1988). The point of departure for a social analysis of medicine is that it comprises not only a very comprehensive and sophisticated set of procedures, but also a body of knowledge, framing a worldview and requiring appropriate socialization, symbolism, and language (Bibeau, 1985; Huizer, 1987; Lepowsky,1990.). In other words, biomedical culture offers its practitioners an accepted way of looking at things. One of its major manifestations is the "medical gaze" (Foucault, 1967), through which the medical profession translates physical and/or mental signs into categories of health, illness, and subsequently treatment (see also Armstrong,1987; Berg, 1995). The medical gaze has been responsible, for example, for the constitution of "madness" as mental illness at the end of the eighteenth century, when "the language of psychiatry, which is a monologue of reason about madness, has been established only on the basis of such a silence" (Foucault, 1967: x).

Good (1994) further illustrates the medical gaze through medical students' descriptions of their learning and socialization process in both the clinical and preclinical years at medical school. The way a student is taught to think "anatomically," shifting the focus from the human being as "a person with an imagined life" to wondering what the person looks like underneath the skin, is a view that demands not only medical but cultural work as well. A common pathway of access to the human body taught at medical school is the microscope. Good's description of the order in which slides are shown at a lecture illuminates this point: "A slide showing the epidemiology of the disease will be followed by a clinical slide of a patient, and then by a pathological specimen. Then a slide of low magnification cell structure is followed by an electron micrograph, and from this level to diagrams of molecular structure and genetic expression" (1994: 75). Biomedicine reduces the entirety of the human body to the cellular level and explains disease through the basic sciences. This is the grand narrative of modern medicine. Against this backdrop, I will later ask whether NCM constructs an alternative reality to that of conventional biomedicine, in which the authoritative doctor–patient relationship is replaced by a more egalitarian dyad, the biological emphasis is supplanted by a holistic mind/body outlook, and disease is treated by concentrating on systemic equilibrium rather than superficial physical symptoms.

The next stage to seeing medically is learning to talk and write medically. These are important skills aimed at imposing a certain kind of order on the disorder of human symptoms. Good (1994) discusses the medical write-up not as a mere record of verbal exchange but as a formative practice, a practice that "shapes talk as much as it reflects it" (p. 77). The write-up constructs a person as a patient, a document, and a project. A student interviewed by Good elaborated on this point:

> You begin to approach the patient with a write-up in mind . . . and so you have all these categories that you need to get filled. Because if you don't do that, you go in, you interact . . . you talk . . . you go back and you realize that you left out this, this and this and you need to go back. And when you go in with the write-up mentally emblazoned in your mind, you're thinking in terms of those categories (1994: 78).

The demand to think in terms of the write-up is in fact one of the socializing processes of medical internship. Students learn what kind of details can make the attending physicians impatient or bored: "They don't want to hear the story of the person. They want to hear the edited version" (Good, 1994: 78). Professional behavior, then, is

> Not to talk with people and learn about their lives and nurture them. You're not there for that. You're a professional and you're trained in interpreting phenomenological descriptions of behavior into physiological and pathophysiological processes. So there's the sense of if you try to really tell people the story of someone, they'd be angry; they'd be annoyed at you because you're missing the point. That's indulgence, sort of. You can have that if you want that when you're in the room with the patient. But don't present that to me. What you need to present to me is the stuff we're going to work on (1994: 78).

Medical discourse therefore is a positivistic (neutral and objective) discourse in which human subjectivity is reduced and translated into technical terms. Waitzkin (1991) took medical constructionism further, showing how the medical profession exercises not only physical but also moral control over patients by ignoring the cues they venture as to the cause and nature of their complaint. In the process of its expansion, biomedicine assumed a dominant and distinct position. This ideology of exclusiveness rejected and did away with competing health paradigms, except for cases in which the local ethnomedicine was resilient enough to adapt to and sometimes even contain biomedicine (Bledsoe and Goubaud, 1985; Lim Tan, 1989).

The procedures of biomedicine have been propagated through textbooks and training, colonizing new territories through modern education, international organizations (such as the WHO), and governmental sponsorship. The expansion of biomedicine often went hand in hand with colonialism and is described by Comaroff as a "technique of civilization" (1993: 315) or by Baer, Singer, and Susser (1997) as part of the services provided to local communities as a humane justification for taking over their lands. In China, for example, even though Chinese medicine is probably the world's oldest body of medical knowledge and tradition dating back some four thousand years, Western medicine gained a strong foothold with the assistance of European and U.S. colonial powers in the nineteenth and early twentieth centuries (Baer et al., 1997). Whereas the globalization of biomedical culture has been part of the modernist project, administered by the nation-state and its agencies (Wallerstein, 1974), the globalization of NCM is driven by new postmodern forces such as consumerism and popular culture. The globalization of NCM, in contrast to that of biomedicine, signifies a process of greater plurality. The world does not necessarily become 'united,' but rather more fragmented and hybridized. The globalization of NCM can by no means assume integration in the naive functionalist sense (Featherstone, 1991; Robertson, 1992) due to two principal reasons. First, biomedicine has not been replaced by the competing NCM, but rather stood its ground, with NCM often adapting to it. Second, NCM itself encompasses a plethora of methods, practices, and treatments that do not embody a common paradigm.

This book focuses on a "reversed" type of globalization, in which the periphery (NCM) impinges on the center (biomedicine). A key concept in my discussion of globalization and the diffusion of global and local cultures is that of domestication, and this book will highlight patterns of domestication of NCM in the Israeli context. In this manner, this book joins a growing list of cultural studies that have rendered the local/global interplay a key scenario of the last decade. Images of domestication, hybridization, glocalization, pidginization, and creolization, all designating synonymous processes, have become central metaphors in the study of the flow of culture (Appadurai and Breckenridge, 1988; Der Derian and Shapiro, 1989; Hannerz, 1989; King, 1991; Wilson and Dissanayake, 1996). On the one hand there are global realities, forms, and processes that permeate national borders, such as Hollywood films, soap operas, package tours, chain stores, department stores and malls, fast-food restaurants, theme parks, and alternative medicine therapies. These global forms seem to be drawing the world into a disturbing commercial sameness. However, social entities, such as nation-states, classes, ethnic groups, and social institutions in general, domesticate these global forms through local preferences and cultural patterns.

Outline of the Book

Broadly speaking, this study sets out to explore patterns by which NCM coexists with the biomedical establishment. The first chapter discusses various approaches that have characterized previous studies of NCM. I then propose a typology of patterns of assimilation and acculturation, used to distinguish between the various processes relevant to the existence of NCM. This typology of assimilation and acculturation is used as a framework for discussing four approaches that have characterized previous studies of NCM. All these approaches presented a dichotomous view of health behavior. Yet must behavior be dichotomous? Findings suggest today that many people can be characterized by dual utilization of NCM and biomedicine. In the framework of this study, I therefore adopt a theoretical conceptualization that does not resort to dichotomous categorization.

Chapter 2 discusses the field in which I conducted my ethnographic research—urban Israel. The unique combination of medico-legal arrangements in Israel along with growing public demand for NCM have led to the development of a domesticated type of NCM practiced in urban clinics, taught in colleges, and disseminated in the media. I suggest that NCM in Israel should be examined as an encounter between the global and the local, in which the periphery (NCM) impinges on the cultural map of the center. NCM in Israel is analyzed in this study so as to highlight the particular organizational pattern of its domestication. My argument, however, is that similar processes of domestication are occurring in other industrial countries, in line with local organizational and medico-legal arrangements.

The subsequent chapters provide empirical evidence of the way in which the domestication of NCM has been taking place in Israel. Chapter 3 concentrates on a hospital-adjacent clinic that provides a variety of NCM treatments and describes the communication between MDs and other practitioners of NCM. Analysis of cases presented at staff meetings shows that biomedicine is predominant in the discourse on health and illness conducted at the clinic and that an "alternative" gaze does not really emerge. This chapter also examines the manner in which the clinic constructs the delivery and supervision of treatment as a biomedical enterprise. Chapter 4 describes the attitudes of the clinic's patients and compares them to patients who have never used any form of NCM. Findings presented in this chapter are of particular interest as they clearly show that many patients were using both methods—CM and NCM—concomitantly, and that no particular profile—sociodemographic or cultural—characterized either group. I conclude the section on the clinic by demonstrating that the quantitative data concerning patients' attitudes underpin the interpretations based on the qualitative, ethnographic findings. In general, it is evident that the delivery of NCM in Israel does not suggest the existence of an "alternative" ideology, but rather that NCM has been domesticated by CM. While forces of consumerism and public demand have speeded the popular dissemination of NCM, the public nevertheless prefers to use NCM under the supervision of biomedicine. For this reason, the exotic elements of NCM have been downplayed and fused with scientific components, creating a hybrid form of medical treatment that is ultimately foreign enough to be fascinating, but also familiar enough not to be disconcerting. This, and not the rejection of biomedicine, is probably what has made NCM so popular, both in Israel and elsewhere.

Chapter 5 analyzes the manner in which NCM is disseminated to the general public by means of articles published in the popular press. In this chapter I illustrate the interprofessional discourse between representatives of nonconventional and conventional medicine as it is conducted on the pages of the daily press. In this capacity, authoritative figures, usually MDs practicing NCM, redefine the concepts of health and illness by subtly undermining conventional medicine and promoting the advantages of NCM. These articles provide an interesting instance of the manner in which an opposition between NCM and

CM is created only to be reconciled within the framework of "complementary" or "integrated" medicine. Chapter 6 illustrates the manner in which NCM is taught in Israeli colleges. This is part of the professionalization of NCM. These colleges combine courses on NCM modalities such as homeopathy, acupuncture, or naturopathy with an extensive curriculum based on conventional science and medicine comprising subjects such as anatomy, physiology, and CPR. One of the more advanced and applied courses in the curriculum teaches students to combine Western diagnostic methods with NCM treatments, creating a hybrid that is both "Eastern" and "Western," "exotic" and "familiar" at once. This practice ignores many of the more esoteric and exotic tenets of NCM theory, thereby rendering it palatable to the Israeli consumer. The conclusion returns to the question of domestication, locating it within broader processes such as consumerism, medical pluralism, and the postmodern body.

Chapter 1

Conceptualizing NCM

The focus on domestication carries novel implications, both theoretical and analytical, for the study of NCM. This emphasis is different from prior conceptualizations that rested on a dichotomous interpretation of either dominance or resistance. The concept of domestication is also different from recent discussions of the 'integration' of NCM. Furthermore, whereas the majority of researchers base their analysis either on questionnaires or interviews, this study offers an ethnography of NCM in the media, the colleges, and the clinics. Rather than concentrating on larger samples or a bird's-eye discussion of the medico-legal system, it is essential, in my view, to understand what happens to NCM when it is taught, practiced, and consumed. It is within the negotiated order of such interactions that the domesticated nature of NCM reveals itself.

Approaches in the History of NCM Research

The history of NCM research can be subsumed under four approaches: tradition versus modernity; limited dissatisfaction with conventional medicine; general dissatisfaction with science and technology; and medical pluralism. I present these approaches in the order of their development and then compare the most recent approach, medical pluralism, to the domestication approach offered in this study.

Modernity versus Tradition

The first and earliest approach in the study of NCM rested on a dichotomy between traditionalism and modernity. For example, studies conducted in developing societies often labored under the belief in the dominance of Western biomedicine. In these studies, the relationship between indigenous forms of healing and Western biomedicine was viewed on a continuum of modernization on which indigenous, traditional medicine occupied the nonmodern pole, and Western biomedicine the modern pole. This approach predicted that a gradual process of modernization would eventually bring about the abandonment of traditional, nonscientific medical practices. The modern-traditional dichotomy can be traced back to classical sociological thought, first and foremost to the modernization perspective. The modernization thesis argued that non-Western "developing" countries are "modernized" by emulating the capitalist structure of Western democracy with its educational, technological, political, and medical systems (Parsons, 1966). This perspective rejected the viability of NCM and saw its retention by traditional groups as a temporary situation.

In this vein, for example, Finkler (1981) suggested that measures of an individual's modernity such as level of education or type of employment could be used to predict the likelihood of resorting to biomedicine or traditional healers. Reciprocity between the two systems at the organizational level was not considered a viable proposition. Haram's (1991) study of traditional Tswana medicine described how doctors at the government biomedical clinic expected traditional healers to refer patients to them, but would not, of course, consider returning the courtesy.

When the phenomenon of NCM was examined in the urban context of developed Western societies, the dichotomous principle persisted and the tendency was to transfer the modernization perspective, which had been employed in the study of traditional societies, to the modern milieu. The reason for this might be that homogeneous ethnic groups served as the targets of these studies. For example, Farge (1977) treated the use of traditional health systems by Mexicans as an indicator of low acculturation into the mainstream of modern American society, while Miller (1990) discussed the weakening of traditional health beliefs in non-Western medicine as a function of acculturation to the host society. Because a synthesis between tradition and modernity was ideologically rejected, dual system use, if and when it existed, was considered a transitional practice abandoned once acculturation had been achieved. This approach was aptly summarized by New (1977): "For the stereotyped, middle-class housewife, going to a physician is perfectly respectable, but going to a *curandero* [traditional healer] would not be. If she took prescription drugs, this would be fine, but if certain herbal teas were found in the kitchen cabinet, she may have to explain and rationalize."

In Israel, studies conducted on the health beliefs of homogeneous populations that had emigrated from North African or Middle Eastern countries and could be characterized by low socioeconomic status, extended families, and adherence to traditional beliefs, tended to adopt the view that these practices were transient. Nudelman (1993), for example, described the traditional healing methods of Ethiopian Jews, while Bilu, in a series of studies (1979; 1980; 1990), compared traditional healing among North African Jews and modern psychological treatment. Utilization of traditional healers was described in these cases as a pattern of behavior that had been prevalent in the country of origin and, as such, was carried over to modern Israel together with other customs that were labeled "traditional." Although these studies are interesting, their specific demographic focus prevents the findings from being of relevance to the explanation of health-seeking practices of a more heterogeneous, less traditional population. The study of health practices of more heterogeneous groups brought about a change in the conceptualization described by the modernization approach that reviews the recourse to NCM as a transitional phase in a process of acculturation, the culmination of which will be ascription to one extreme of the modern-traditional sequence.

However, once studies conducted on heterogeneous population groups produced demographic data that indicated that consumers of NCM came from all sectors of society, dual use of different medical systems was no longer viewed as a transient element, nor as a measure of an individual's modernity. The new approach explained recourse to NCM as a measure of an individual's satisfaction with the outcome of treatment received in the framework of conventional medicine. Dissatisfaction with conventional medicine could be limited to a specific form of treatment or medical problem, or could be directed toward the entire system of modern biomedicine. While limited dissatisfaction with conventional medicine labored under the assumption of the hegemony of biomedicine, this tenet was not necessarily embraced by the general dissatisfaction approach. Both approaches, however, believed in a dichotomous divide between the various modalities of NCM and biomedicine.

The "Second Resort" Approach—Limited Dissatisfaction

The realization that explanatory models could not be transferred from low development societies or culturally homogeneous groups within high development societies to the more heterogeneous fabric of modern, Western society led to a different sort of conceptualization. I call this approach the "second resort" approach. Like the "modernization approach," the second resort approach also assumed the hegemonic status of Western, scientific medicine. Departing from the confines of biomedicine was viewed as feasible only after a particular health problem had not been solved. The recourse to an "irrational" option such as NCM could then be constructed, in effect, as rational behavior.

A study conducted by Ronen (1988) in Israel showed that the use of NCM in Israel was not limited to a subgroup characterized by a specific ethnic background, low income, or low level of education. At the outset, Ronen indeed labored under the assumption that

> In relation to people who utilize this type of treatment [NCM], general opinion is that, on the whole, they are 'simple,' uneducated, mostly from lower classes of society, not over-discerning, and prepared to adopt various beliefs without adequate scientific foundation making it easy to persuade them to try such kinds of treatment (1998: 17).

At the conclusion of his study, however, Ronen was forced to express "surprise" that consumers of NCM came from all levels of income and education. His conclusion was that recourse to NCM should be viewed as a "functional alternative" to conventional medicine—functional in the sense that it is limited to the attempt to solve a specific medical problem and does not reflect a comprehensive ideology, outlook, or lifestyle.

This position was also evident in studies in the same period by Kronenfeld and Wasner (1982), Gray (1985), and Goldstein (1988). These studies were conducted among patients suffering from chronic diseases such as rheumatoid arthritis or asthma and findings generally indicated that patients usually first sought help from an MD. However, when the problem was not solved by conventional medicine because the disease was chronic or recurrent, patients found it legitimate to turn to NCM. In an early work, Sharma (1992), too, did not view the increased resort to NCM as evidence of an important cultural shift in thinking about health, the person, or the body. She claimed that users of NCM were impelled by a pragmatic concern to get relief from a disease.

General Dissatisfaction—New Age Challenges to Biomedical Hegemony

An additional group of studies conducted on the use of NCM in the modern context suggested that the growing popularity of NCM in healing, as well as health maintenance, reflected a more generalized dissatisfaction with conventional medicine. This general dissatisfaction or disenchantment has been labeled "postmodern" by some commentators (Lyotard, 1987). From this perspective, the clients of NCM could be characterized as not being in the process of modernization, but in the process of rejecting modernity. For example, in a study conducted by Cant and Calnan (1991), one nonconventional practitioner is quoted as saying that for 20% of her patients she served as a first resort for primary care since they had adopted a "natural lifestyle." This approach can be seen to have replaced the "modern versus traditional" dichotomy with that of "West versus East" or "familiar versus exotic." Furthermore, placing NCM as part of a more general, postmodern "counterculture" implied a process of demedicalization driven by a consumerist quest for alternative treatments and individual philosophies of health maintenance.

Whereas the limited dissatisfaction approach viewed NCM as "second resort," the general dissatisfaction approach viewed NCM as "counterculture." NCM use was equated with ideological concern for ecology (Bakx, 1991), preoccupation with the body (Glassner, 1989), and fascination with the cultural "other" and the supernatural. Once more a dichotomy is implied between established and dissident cultural forms. Lupton (1994), for example, saw NCM as offering a "solution to the growing domination of high technology with all its impersonality" because "most alternative therapies eschew the use of high technology and lab reports in diagnosing and treating illness and disease."

Mary Douglas (1994) has proven a noteworthy proponent of the view that recourse to NCM should be seen as part of a countercultural movement. According to Douglas, NCM is "alternative in the full countercultural sense, 'spiritual' in contrast to 'material,' " and provides a "cultural alternative to western philosophic traditions." Douglas explained that

> When the same population is divided in its adherence to one or the other world view, cultural conflict is present. As the people hear the themes of the conflict, competition between cultural principles spreads; soon no one will be able to stay neutral as to meat eating, or religion, or concern for the environment. Even medicine may be a ground for testing allegiance (1994: 25).

Douglas contends that "it is important to appreciate that a person cannot, for long, belong to two cultures at once" and assumes the existence of a coherent cultural type, arguing that "we would expect people who show a strong preference for holistic medicine to be negative to the kind of culture in which the other kind of medicine belongs. If they have made the choice for gentler, more spiritual medicine, they will be making the same choice in other contexts, dietary, ecological, as well as medical. The choice of holistic medicine will not be an isolated preference, uncoordinated with other values upheld by the patient" (p. 32). Douglas therefore extends the scope of dichotomies, suggesting that not only must behavior in the medical sphere entail choice, but that this choice will automatically lead to more inclusive and extensive dichotomies.

Medical Pluralism

Many recent studies on recourse to NCM have shown that patients tend to adopt a pluralistic approach to health care and move with facility from conventional medicine to nonconventional medicine and also from one nonconventional modality to another, according to necessity. Seen in the framework of medical pluralism, health-seeking consumerist activity is no longer regarded as "dissatisfaction with conventional medicine" (second approach) or as "cultural rebellion" (third approach). According to the approach called medical pluralism, people seek nonconventional health treatments to maximize their prospects for quality of life. They are 'smart consumers' who make full use of the range of health therapies available in the market. This approach argues that the majority of health consumers use both conventional medicine and NCM concomitantly. Several studies conducted in different parts of the world such as Canada, Australia, the United States, and England have provided data that support this claim (Cant and Sharma, 1996;

Kelner and Wellman, 1997; McGregor and Peay, 1996; McGuire, 1988; Sirois and Gick, 2002).

Cant and Sharma's (1999) analysis of "medical pluralism" in the United Kingdom focuses on "pluralistic legitimation" and "therapeutic divergence"—a multiple coexistence of methods (e.g., homeopathy, Chinese medicine, chiropractic, and so on) side by side with biomedicine. In their conclusion, the authors contend that the recognition of certain therapies as 'legitimate' has meant that the state has been increasingly prepared to legislate accreditation; however, "recognition has only been granted where therapy groups have undergone a process of 'convergence' with biomedicine" (Cant and Sharma, 1999: 186). A parallel discussion of the status of a variety of heterodox medical systems in the United States is provided by Baer (2001) who offers an extensive list of the states in which each modality is licensed and suggests that licensing often entails compatibility with the biomedical model of organization (118).

In addition to the approach of medical pluralism, I would like to suggest another perspective to the study of NCM—that of domestication. In this process the philosophical tenets of treatment modalities that differ from the explanatory and diagnostic modes of biomedicine are modified and culturally translated. These modalities are rendered more culturally acceptable and less exotic, foreign, and ultimately challenging. The growing popularity of NCM modalities and the facility with which individuals move from biomedicine to nonconventional medicine, illustrated by the approach of "medical pluralism," can most probably be explained by the domestication of these modalities in the image of biomedicine. In this manner culturally foreign treatments seem feasible and make sense to patients from a cultural point of view. McGuire (1988), for example, has shown how modalities such as shiatsu, chiropractic, acupuncture, and reflexology have lost much of their ritualistic tenor, becoming more of a technique. McGuire argues that in this case the technique itself, and not the beliefs supporting it, seems to be the key attraction for most adherents. Barnes (1998) and Hare (1993) have also explored processes by which Chinese medicine delivered in the United States has been tailored to American needs and expectations.

Although the high incidence of nonconventional therapies and techniques could create the impression of medical pluralism, NCM has not gained equal status to biomedicine, in Israel and elsewhere, as the term "medical pluralism" would imply. Rather, its successful incorporation into the therapeutic repertoire of developed countries has proved to depend, in principle, on biomedical approval and the imitation of biomedical symbols, terminology, and professional practice. The medical pluralism approach does not dwell much on the role of cultural commitment in the choice of health care, putting down these choices to pragmatic consumerism. My claim is that medicine must make sense to patients, and this feat requires cultural domestication. The counterculture approach, which does emphasize the cultural dimension of NCM, cannot explain the facility with which patients move between NCM and biomedicine as it presumes deep commitment to a specific worldview. On the other hand, the approach of medical pluralism ignores the issue of cultural acceptability. The question to be answered is how patients move among the various modalities, make sense of them at least in a perfunctory, superficial manner, and find them culturally acceptable?

Domestication: Making Sense of Medicine

In a discussion of the fit between cultural context and medical treatment, McQueen (1985) contends that the interest in Chinese systems of medicine waned in the United States after its popularity peaked in the 1970s. The reason for this decline in popularity was due, according to McQueen, to the ultimate unacceptability of the Chinese model in Western society. The author explained that culture, like a biological species, adapts to a particular niche in the ecology and is rarely, if ever, directly transplantable from one society or ecological environment to another. In the long run, however, McQueen's conclusions proved to be mistaken. In 1993, Eisenberg et al. published a widely quoted study in *The New England Journal of Medicine*, presenting figures that indicated that not only was the utilization of Chinese medicine widespread in the United States (among other forms of NCM), but that it was also a lucrative business.

The contemporary consumption of NCM points to a flaw in McQueen's discussion of NCM as an idea without context and therefore a misfit in American society. Something must have happened in the interim to explain the fallacy of McQueen's interpretation. If Chinese medicine continued to gain popularity, then ideas planted in unfamiliar niches could, in fact, flourish. This leads to two alternative explanations. First, the unfamiliarity of NCM could have become a source of attraction. This explanation continues the reasoning of "difference" that has been developed by the general dissatisfaction/counterculture view. Second, NCM may have been contextualized and better adapted to its new niche. This explanation points toward acculturation and domestication, the focus of this study.

Discussing the consumption of a domesticated form of Chinese medicine in Western society, Unschuld (1987) explains the popularity of Chinese medicine in the West through the parameter of 'inauthenticity.' He claims that

> Throughout the USA and Europe *so-called* Chinese medicine is practiced and finds a clientele of patients. Mostly, though, this 'Chinese medicine' is limited to acupuncture and to certain notions of health, illness and therapeutic intervention that often enough appear to mirror western ideas of what 'alternative' medicine should be like, rather than original Chinese thought.

Unschuld suggests that in the search for an Asian alternative, the basic values of Western civilization were applied to select from a heterogeneous bundle of concepts and practices those that appeared plausible to a Western audience. Unschuld discussed, for example, the culturally biased translation of a Chinese concept (*qi*) as "energy." According to him, the more exact term would be closer to the word "vapor," something like light tiny drops of matter, which has evaporated.

Unschuld's observations are supported by other studies. Barnes (1998), in a study of the indigenizing of Chinese healing practices in the American context, claims that the language of "energy blockages" used in American Chinese healing imitates popular American psychology that describes an individual as "blocked" or "stuck." This reflects domestication to American norms since it caters to the American need to externalize, discuss, and explain emotions, practices that would be considered deviant in a Chinese context. In order to find "authentic" Chinese treatments for psychological problems, American acupuncturists are going back to ancient Chinese texts and retrieving portions that had been deleted by the Chinese authorities in the "cultural revolution" because they were considered magic and religious and therefore "unscientific." According to Barnes (1998), this represents the cultural reinterpretation of "Chinese medicine" in American eyes. In her apt words, "What looks back at us remains Chinese medicine, but now wears a distinctly American face" (Barnes, 1998: 438).

Observing a consultation between a practitioner of traditional Chinese medicine and a Chinese patient in Taiwan, Kleinman (1980) describes an encounter that lasted for less than two minutes. The practitioner registered the patient's chief complaint, took his pulse (a form of diagnosis in ancient Chinese medicine), and wrote a prescription. This technical transaction was a far cry from the holistic and philosophical style in which "traditional Chinese medicine" is represented in the West. It appears that, in its original location, traditional Chinese medicine can be overtly technical because there is no need to philosophize with patients about "energy." The philosophy is already taken for granted, and part of the common cultural heritage of physicians and patients. Kleinman's observations are especially pertinent when examined along with the following observation made by a Chinese practitioner working with an American clientele:

> The whole relationship with patients is different. Here the patients seem to want to know more about what you are going to do, the components of the herbs and their side effects. In China people don't ask because they already know. It is part of their background even if it is the first time they are going to see a practitioner. Also Chinese people are not tending to ask questions. They don't ask why (Barnes, 1998: 420).

Studies such as these conducted by Unschuld, Barnes, and Kleinman show that Chinese medicine practiced in the West is selective and mirrors Western ideas of plausibility, and that the West constructs images of Oriental medicine. This brings to mind the work of Edward Said (1978) on Orientalism. We are standing at an important junction where positivistic claims regarding the "authentic" are replaced by postpositivist, interpretive arguments concerning mirroring and representation.

This fusion of the foreign and the familiar to produce a locally acceptable hybrid is a process that has also been observed when the center impinges on the periphery as in the case of Western, biomedicine becoming part of low development countries. For example, studies conducted in low development societies have shown how antibiotics have been used according to the color of the capsule in order to incorporate them into the categorization of diseases as hot or cold (Bledsoe and Goubaud, 1985). Another study involving African chemists in South Africa has shown how traditional herbs were packaged to resemble biomedical OTC pharmaceuticals but retained their culturally relevant African brand names and motifs (Cocks and Dold, 2000). This is the same process that occurs when nonscientific modalities, those called alternative or complementary therapies, are introduced into high development, industrialized societies when the more esoteric parts of these modalities are played down in order to gain acceptance (Baer, 1998; 2001; Dew, 2000). According to Hare (1993: 38), "one of the most striking aspects of the incorporation of the Chinese medical systems into western health care is the degree to which there is a mixing of classical Chinese, other scholarly or professional east Asian, and modern Chinese medical thought, with a variety of folk paradigms from east Asia, and the many ethnic streams of the western locale in which the new 'Oriental' medicine is now being practiced." All these examples entail a process of "making sense of medicine," which is effected through the creation of local hybrid forms. This is the domestication that, I argue, serves as a prerequisite to practices of pluralistic consumption.

Acculturation and Assimilation

In order to understand the various stages and processes inherent in the interface between conventional biomedicine and nonconventional medicine, I will suggest a schematic model that organizes these processes on two dimensions: assimilation and acculturation.

This model was originally proposed by Hood and Koberg (1994) to describe the adaptation of nondominant minority groups to dominant majority groups in organizations. Indeed, contact between cultures has often been studied through the dimensions of acculturation and assimilation. McElroy and Townsend (1989: 297), for example, define acculturation as "continuous contact between two previously autonomous cultural traditions, usually leading to extensive changes in one or both systems." Assimilation, on the other hand, occurs when the minority group becomes a normative component of the dominant society. Assimilation is not merely a consummation of acculturation, but an independent axis. The typology of assimilation and acculturation can thus provide a framework for organizing previous NCM research. Furthermore, the changes that NCM has undergone in the course of its integration can be conceived as a specific path of movement from one category to another within the matrix of the model. This complements my claim that domestication is a dynamic process.

NCM's introduction into Western countries is comparable with the absorption of immigrants into a different society or country, a process variously described by anthropologists and sociologists in crosscultural research as adaptation, acculturation, or assimilation (Berry, 1990; Berry,

Kim, and Boski, 1988; McElroy and Townsend, 1989). In a similar manner, NCM is a "stranger" in the Western world of biomedicine, caught on the margin between two cultures—its original ideology and the host culture of biomedicine. Such marginality can be resolved through acculturation and assimilation.

The proposed model suggests a fourfold categorization of the statuses and roles of the "newcomer" minority group according to differing levels of acculturation and assimilation. Figure 1 illustrates the contact between the dominant (biomedical) culture and the adapting group (NCM). In studies of cultural contact it is customary to assess the difference between the two cultures by examining behaviors and belief systems in their traditional, pre-contact form, and then comparing them to the post-contact situation. The cultural features of the group, once adapted, may not be the same as those of the original group on first contact. With continued contact the groups and the individuals within them continue to change. In the case of NCM, we are interested not only in the post-contact form but also the original form. As a result of acculturation or assimilation, NCM can change its original form, becoming integrated, domesticated, or differentiated in the process.

Acculturation changes the nondominant group's cultural patterns and behaviors to those of a dominant group or society; it requires the nondominant group to "take on" and learn the culture of the dominant group. Assimilation, by contrast, is the acceptance of a nondominant group (or individual members of it) by mainstream society. In the case of NCM, the major factor behind assimilation is public demand. Established biomedicine cannot, in principle, accept or assimilate NCM, which it regards as nonscientific and hence ex-paradigmatic. The ac-

	High **Acculturation** *Low*	
High	Domestication	Differentiation
Assimilation		
Low	Selective integration	Rejection

Figure 1. Patterns of assimilation and acculturation.

ceptance of NCM practitioners into professional organizations, hospital clinics, medical school programs, and other institutions of mainstream society depends on the good will of biomedicine and usually occurs in response to public demand. Since NCM addresses the public independently through the media, forces of consumption may well generate a demand for NCM even under the gaze of biomedicine. I will deal with biomedical influence on the acculturation of NCM in the chapter on the complementary clinic, where NCM practitioners are partially and conditionally assimilated by working under the supervision of physicians. The public factor behind assimilation will be analyzed in the chapter on patients and their attitudes, as well as in the chapter on NCM in the media. My overall findings suggest that biomedical supervision and public demand have become entangled in NCM. For example, whereas NCM colleges and clinics might have been established in response to public demand, biomedicine retained its influence in these institutions.

In many cases, some degree of acculturation is necessary for assimilation to occur, although the opposite may also exist—for example, in the case of a counterculture, when a social group embraces an antiestablishment or alternative behavior. In such a case, the minority culture gains public popularity (assimilation) without altering its original form in order to be more like the host culture (acculturation). Some degree of assimilation can facilitate acculturation, since certain behaviors and values involving power and negotiation are often deliberately hidden from those outside the powerful group. As processes, acculturation and assimilation constitute an interactive system. In this capacity it is important to recognize the relative power of different sectors of the public and their potential influence on the medical establishment. For example, it might be relatively easy for the medical establishment to marginalize the practices of weaker, less influential groups in society, such as immigrants or migrant workers. However, the involvement of established, middle-class individuals in the practice and consumption of NCM and their demand for such services might be more difficult to ignore. It is also important to point out that the medical establishment should not be perceived as a heterogeneous group concerning its stand on NCM. While there are indeed MDs who practice NCM and GPs who refer patients to NCM practitioners (Perkin et al., 1994; White et al., 1997), many senior members of the medical profession who serve on political and professional committees often marginalize and reject NCM altogether.

Both acculturation and assimilation may be measured on continua, but for purposes of conceptual presentation, the two dimensions can be treated as falling into two categories—high and low. The result is a fourfold classification in which each cell represents a different pattern of adaptation: *domestication, selective integration, differentiation, and rejection* (see Fig. 1). These four patterns evidently represent ideal types. The course of development of NCM and the relevant approaches to its study can now be described in the following manner, using the concepts that appear in Figure 1.

The first encounter, more than thirty years ago, between biomedicine and NCM began in the lower right cell, where the low assimilation and low acculturation of NCM resulted in its *rejection*. This encounter took place when ethnic groups, usually immigrants, continued to practice their traditional medicine even though they were living in a modern, industrial context in which biomedicine was hegemonic. This situation represented the rejection of NCM (conceived as traditional) by biomedicine (conceived as modern). The first approach to the study of NCM, which regards the relationship between NCM and biomedicine within the dichotomy of tradition versus modernity, belongs to the category of rejection.

Public demand (responsible for growing assimilation) and biomedical hegemony (responsible for growing acculturation) were the major factors that drove NCM out of 'rejection' and into the nearby cells of 'differentiation' and 'selective integration.' The second approach to the study of NCM emphasized it as a 'second resort' owing to patients' dissatisfaction with the results of conventional medical treatments. This approach leads to *selective integration*. According to this approach, NCM attracts pragmatic people who seek treatment for a specific condition that was not treated successfully by conventional medicine. From a diachronic point of view, the low assimilation of NCM in this approach can be explained by its adoption by specific and select segments of the population and the medical profession. This can be illustrated, for example, when an MD uses an NCM modality that has not gained public popularity. The option of domestication, which is characterized not only by high acculturation, as in the case of selective integration, but also by high assimilation, occurred much later when NCM became increasingly popular with large sectors of the public. In this capacity it was perceived as one more option on the health market as outlined in the fourth approach, that of pluralism.

The third approach regards NCM as a cultural alternative, and those who seek it as cultural rebels. This approach represents low acculturation, since NCM does not attempt to mold itself into biomedical patterns. A rising public demand for such NCM treatments represents high assimilation. This combination of low acculturation and high assimilation brings NCM into a state of *differentiation*. The differentiated NCM is not domesticated. On the contrary, its raison d'etre is an emphasis on the essential and critical difference from conventional medicine. NCM methods such as crystals or Reiki can thus be popular and still maintain esoteric philosophical characteristics.

The fourth approach, medical pluralism, developed as both the acculturation and assimilation of NCM were on the rise. This approach regards NCM patients as smart consumers seeking to maximize their options in the health market. This approach is relevant to *domestication*. It is yet to be seen whether NCM will be taking any one prominent direction in the future, and which direction it will be.

Domestication and the Flow of Culture

I argue that the key to understanding the success of NCM can be found in the ways in which it has been domesticated or hybridized (Baer, 2001; Hannerz, 1992, 1996). In a parallel manner to Tobin's definition of domestication (1992: 4), the changes of NCM should be understood as "a process that is active (unlike westernization, modernization, or postmodernism), morally neutral (unlike imitation or parasitism), and demystifying (there is nothing inherently strange, exotic, or unique going on around here)."

A question often raised in regard to domestication is whether the process in which the exotic is rendered familiar actually results in the "other," forgoing its claim to uniqueness. Bauman (1992a) suggested that the extensive fragmentation of modern culture might indicate the absence of a fixed point of reference from which "self" and "other" can be defined. The nonexistence of a recognized mainstream would therefore preclude the existence of an alternative. Turner (1994) has pointed out that a new level of multiculturalism has emerged from globalization that posed a challenge to many of the traditional dominant cultures of nation-states. Said (1993: 15) illustrated the same point by asking: "Who in India or Algeria today can confidently separate out the British or

French component of the past from present actualities, and who in Britain or France can draw a clear circle around British London or French Paris that would exclude the impact of India or Algeria upon these two imperial cities?" The notion that "otherness has been domesticated" (Turner, 1994: 183) could in fact lead to a general sense of fitting in. However, the postmodern predicament of domestication seems to have propagated a sense of alienation and loneliness. The predominant sentiment is that of being a "stranger at home," rather than the sense of belonging to a community and developing communal bonds. In the absence of a center, the individual is forced into continual reflexivity and questioning of authenticity.

This sense of being a stranger at home has triggered a nostalgic quest for community and for "things as they used to be." I suggest that the growing popularity of NCM, in its domesticated forms, is part of this quest. NCM treatments are conceived by many as a personalized and intimate alternative in contrast to the alienating, technological anonymity of biomedical health care. Moreover, the body has become a primary locus of individual control and self-realization, providing a metaphoric dwelling for the "homeless mind" of the postmodern tourist. Much sociological discussion has recently explored the central place that trends such as body building, exercise, cosmetic surgery, and other practices of tending the body have come to occupy in our lives. We have indeed become "pilgrims of the body." Hannerz (1996: 27), for example, remarked that "If there is now a growing celebration in social and cultural theory of the body as a symbolic site of self and continuity, and of the senses, a greater concern with the body and the senses in their contexts might help us understand what 'place' is about." Similarly, Turner (1994: 190) argued that "in contemporary society the body has become a site of regulative beliefs and practices which help to constitute the body as a project." In Shilling's (1993) view, the unfinished project of the self has become converted into the (equally endless) project of the body. All this has meant good business for NCM treatments and practices, which are popularly represented as naturalistic and holistic. One of the goals of the following ethnography is to describe the practice of NCM as one more project of the body within postmodern consumer culture. In its public discourse, NCM portrays the body as a potential site of individual empowerment and purification, at the same time subjecting it to further regulation and control in a manner that reproduces and extends the medical gaze. The imagery and regulation of the body disseminated by NCM are therefore also pertinent to the study of its domestication.

Chapter 2

Setting the Scene: NCM in Israel

A number of historic processes and cultural preferences have given rise to the variations in the relative popularity of specific NCM modalities in European countries (Fisher and Ward, 1994) and in different states in America (Baer, 2001; Van Hemel, 2001). For example, osteopathy, chiropractic, and acupuncture are particularly popular in the United States, homeopathy in England and France, and herbalism and homeopathy in Germany. In contrast, NCM in Israel constitutes a relatively undifferentiated entity, due to various factors connected with the nation-building process. Although the population of Israel is made up of immigrants from a score of different countries and cultures such as Europe, Asia, and Northern Africa, much of the cultural heritage of these very different groups was discarded as irrelevant due to official government policy in the 1950s and 1960s (Lissak and Hurowitz, 1989). In the nation-building days of the State of Israel, the official ideology was that of a "melting pot," and the government conducted an orchestrated and conscious attempt to create a "new Jew" devoid of the signs and symbols of the diaspora. Whereas the "old Jew" was associated with weakness and persecution, the new Jewish society being formed was socialist, secular, and rational, and emphasized the collective at the expense of the individual.

Zionist ideology caused a break in the natural continuity of the flow of culture from one generation to another and parts of the parents' culture were scorned and discarded by the younger generation (Zerubavel, 1996). Cultural practices from the land of origin were called "diasporic" (*galuti*), which is a denigrating description for anything that was not Israeli. In this manner, language, dress, literature, and music as well as informal medical beliefs and practices were not passed on from one generation to the next. Since many of the modalities parceled up in the basket of NCM available in Israel today—such as homeopathy, reflexology, chiropractic, or herbalism—originated in the immigrants' land of origin, they were all initially delegitimized. When public demand increased the popularity of NCM, these different methods were perceived as belonging to the same exotic category as Indian Ayur Vedah and Chinese acupuncture.

The integration of different NCM modalities into one seemingly homogenous category can be linked to additional factors. First, all these modalities are based on theories of illness and disease that differ paradigmatically from that of biomedicine. This explanation is not to be taken lightly as use of all these modalities and the belief in their efficacy constitute an epistemic break in the belief in science and evidence-based medicine as the only basis for treatment. In addition to being rejected as "diasporic," NCM was therefore also rejected for not being in line with the biomedicine that the new State was making every effort to provide on a national and socialistic basis to all its citizens. Furthermore, the acute and epidemiological nature of the health problems that had to be dealt with during the 1950s and 1960s—such as cholera, typhus, malaria, polio, tuberculosis, and malnutrition—were best handled by biomedicine (Shvarts, 2000). Moreover, many children grew up apart from their parents in boarding schools, kibbutzim, or agricultural youth villages. Others arrived in Israel without their parents. For all these reasons, NCM emerged in Israel at a relatively late stage and without cultural continuity. Therefore, second- and third-generation Israelis using NCM are equally unfamiliar with modalities originating either in the West or the East. There can be no validity in Israel to the claim raised in other countries that various strands of medical treatments developed alongside biomedicine. The official medicine of Israel was collective, it was unified, and it was biomedicine (Shuval and Anson, 2000).

An exception to this general state of affairs can be witnessed in the practices of one large group—immigrants from Islamic and North African countries. These immigrants were usually settled in rural, homogeneous communities and therefore preserved their folk medicine along with other cultural practices. For these communities, healing was often combined with religious functions and frequently performed by a religious figure (Bilu, 1977; Palgi, 1978). This type of medicine was called traditional medicine and it was expected to disappear along with acculturation into mainstream Israeli society.

Following the nation-building ethos of the early days of the State of Israel in the 1950s and 1960s, Israeli society has undergone a process of individualization (for discussions of this issue by Israeli sociologists see Eisenstadt, 1985; Katriel, 1986, 1991; Katz and Gurevitch, 1976; Lissak and Hurowitz, 1989; Zerubavel, 1995). The collective ideology has been largely abandoned and many of the last stalwarts of collectivism such as the kibbutz are undergoing a process of privatization. From a cultural point of view this process has been delineated by a revival of interest in traditional and ethnic practices and customs that were set aside due to the melting-pot ideology. From the point of view of medical treatment, in addition to the growing popularity of imported NCM modalities, there has been a reemergence in interest in traditional medicine often combined with religious purposes. This can been observed in pilgrimages to the graves of Jewish rabbis considered miracle-makers (*tzaddikim*), prayer meetings, and wearing amulets. Such activities can be viewed as part of a local display of New Age interest in mysticism or spirituality. From a socioanthropological point of view, they are also connected to the social mobility of specific ethnic groups in Israel (Bilu and Ben-Ari, 1992). It is important, however, to point out that these religious healing practices have not become part of the basket of institutionalized NCM treatments offered in Israel.

NCM in all its forms is therefore a relatively new phenomenon in Israeli society, due to the unique history of Israel in general and that of the establishment of health services in particular. Israeli society provides an example of the cultural negotiation surrounding NCM, which is being conducted in a paradoxical context. Whereas the hegemonic status of biomedicine in Israel has resulted in strict legislation against nonconventional medical practice, these laws are not enforced and are, in fact, widely infringed. NCM treatments in Israel have therefore become subjected to unofficial regulation influenced by market forces.

The Legal Status of NCM in Israel

The National Health Insurance Law, which came into effect January 1, 1995, entitles every Israeli citizen to a wide range of medical services by one of the four health insurance organizations and some 8.7% of Israel's GNP is allocated to health, similar to the level among Western industrialized countries (Grinstein et al., 2002). Nevertheless, as in other Western societies, Israel has recently experienced a rise in the activity of and demand for NCM (Bernstein and Shuval, 1997). A nationwide survey conducted in 1993 in Israel by the Brandman Institute focused on individuals over the age of eighteen and showed that in one-fifth of the households surveyed, one family member had sought out NCM treatment in the course of the previous year. A more recent survey conducted by the Maccabi HMO (the second largest HMO in Israel) showed that 30% of the population in Israel had used NCM (*Ha'aretz* 19.10.2000). An additional survey conducted by the Admati Research Institute for "Medicin" NCM College among 1,131 respondents found that 45% of the Israeli population had received NCM treatment (*Ma'ariv* 10.7.2002). In the United States, in comparison, 42.1% are said to have consulted at least one NCM practitioner during 1997, and paid $10.3 billion out-of-pocket for unconventional care (Eisenberg et al., 1998).

Due to the growing popularity and availability of NCM in Israel a twelve-member committee, headed by former deputy president of the Supreme Court, Menachem Eilon, was formed in 1988 to look into the issue of NCM. The committee's task was to investigate whether NCM modalities could be recognized by the state, and who should be licensed to treat patients with these modalities. The need for the committee was quite acute as no prior legislation in Israel existed concerning the supervision of NCM treatments and practitioners. Indeed, the law regulating the practice of medicine in Israel (the doctor's order of 1976) limited the treatment of individuals to MDs only. Clause 1 of the order defines "the practice of medicine" as "examining patients and injured persons, diagnosing and healing them, writing prescriptions, supervising pregnancy and childbirth or other services generally rendered by a doctor including treatment with acupuncture." Clause 2 defines an authorized doctor as an individual who has a license to practice medicine in accordance with the doctor's order. Clause 3 stipulates that whoever has not been licensed in accordance with the terms of the order will not practice medicine, and will not represent himself either explicitly or implicitly as a practitioner of medicine. In view of the stipulations of this order, there is no provision for treatment, diagnosis or healing of patients outside of the medical profession. It is interesting to note that acupuncture is mentioned in the doctor's order as a modality that can be practiced by licensed MDs only.

The Eilon Committee Report for the Investigation of Complementary Medicine in Israel was subsequently filed in September 1991 and based its recommendations on testimonies gathered from expert witnesses specializing in NCM, conventional MDs, and experience gathered in countries abroad. Legislative practices existing in other countries were also considered by the committee.

In its report the committee stated that it would have preferred to link the licensing of NCM practice with scientific evidence concerning its efficacy. However, the fact that many Israelis were consuming and practicing NCM ruled out this possibility and called for immediate formulation of regulatory policy. The legal situation concerning the practice of NCM in Israel is described in the committee's report as "far from satisfactory." No legal status existed for NCM practitioners who were in fact breaking the law and were, strictly speaking, liable for punishment. Moreover, guidelines did not exist concerning the scope or nature of the professional training of these practitioners and the range of problems they were allowed to deal with. The committee therefore expressed concern that patients might potentially be harmed by infection with hepatitis due to use of unsterilized acupuncture needles or delay of conventional treatment due to misdiagnosis, charlatanism, and cheating.

In its recommendations the committee drew on three fundamental principles in Israeli society. A balance had to be reached between the first two principles—the freedom of choice of medical treatment, and the concern for public safety. In the interest of public safety, when harm was a possibility, the committee felt that treatment should only be administered by a licensed MD. On the other hand, patients should be allowed to exercise freedom of choice and therefore treatment in the framework of complementary medicine should be permitted and not constitute a breach of law. In this manner a third basic principle in Israeli society was upheld—the freedom of occupation and earning a living.

It is interesting to note at this point that the committee refers to NCM as a basket of treatments under the heading "complementary" medicine and singles out the factor of "potential harm" as the primary deciding factor whether treatment should be administered by an MD or a non-MD practitioner. Based on this rationale, the committee then spelled out the very fundamental changes in Israeli legislation it was recommending. The committee stated that the three fundamental principles on which it based its recommendations were acceptable in "other civilized countries" as well as in the State of Israel.

The subsequent recommendations were that:

1. The law should define activities solely limited to MDs, such as diagnosis, prescribing medications, granting sick leave certificates, and treating the mentally ill.

2. Minors can only be treated by NCM after first being treated by an MD and referred by him or her.

3. Any practitioner who is not a doctor must not use the title doctor unless the specific nature of the degree is noted in order to prevent confusion with MDs. Moreover, the initials ND (naturopathic doctor) or OMD (oriental medical doctor) are not to be used in order to prevent confusion among the public.

4. Licensing of various NCM modalities will not be discussed because of the vast differences that exist among these modalities. The committee felt that the time was not yet ripe to define requirements for the licensing, recognition, and supervision of each and every NCM modality on an individual basis and for this reason the Ministry of Health could not be expected to recognize these occupations and supervise their licensing. The task of the Ministry of Health was to concentrate on protecting the public from potential damage and misconception. The practice of complementary medicine should therefore be permitted subject to the limitations previously mentioned according to the legal principles existing in Britain. This called for the establishment of professional registeries supervised by NCM professionals and not necessarily MDs. In the framework of measures required to protect the public, it was suggested that the Ministry of Health adopt legislative practices similar to those existing in Sweden that stipulate that a non-MD practitioner who caused harm to a patient subsequent to treatment should be punished in line with a clause "charlatanism leading to damage to health." It was hoped that the supervision of training and licensing of NCM practitioners by NCM professional organizations would provide a solution to the current problem in Israel where a growing number of individuals were practicing various complementary medicine modalities without satisfactory or sufficient training. To fulfill this purpose, the professional organizations of NCM would have to be invested with the power to oversee training and this would hopefully culminate in future guidelines concerning the recognition of the various modalities, baselines

for professional expertise, and the development of a core of professional ethics.

The committee foresaw a situation in which, following development of uniform programs of training, systematic evaluation of practitioners' knowledge and skills, and proof of efficacy of treatment, the Ministry of Health would recognize and register certain modalities as health professions. It was stressed, however, that the recommendations made by the committee for regulation and supervision of NCM should not be viewed as recognition of the scientific value of complementary medicine.

Homeopathic medications that were currently forbidden for sale in Israel would be permitted for marketing as long as they appeared in the homeopathic pharmacopeia in the United States or Europe and bore the label "the Ministry of Health certifies that this remedy is non-toxic; however, there is no proof of its efficacy." The committee also expressed concern about the widespread advertising of NCM modalities and practitioners in the press that could mislead the public. It was recommended that the same laws that prevent MDs from advertising themselves should be applied to all branches of complementary medicine.

Not all members of the committee agreed with these recommendations, which were indeed controversial concerning the medical profession's hegemonic and exclusive status in the treatment of patients, and a minority opinion was published together with the committee's recommendations. This addendum reflected the views of two senior physicians and a lawyer who represented the Ministry of Health on the committee. This opinion basically stated that Israeli society was not yet ready for such a basic change in law. It contended that the arrangements viable in England concerning the supervision of NCM practice were not transferable to the Israeli milieu. England has a well-established tradition of professional ethics and professional registers have existed there for hundreds of years. Israeli society was not considered mature enough for this type of regulation in view of the current situation in which even the existence of an explicit clause in the law forbidding the practice of medicine by non-MDs was impossible to enforce. Revoking this law would bring about a situation of complete loss of control in which charlatanism and misconduct would flourish at the expense of an innocent public. The duty to protect the public from harm thus outweighed, in this case, the freedom of occupation and freedom to choose medical treatment. The minority report therefore recommended that only scientifically proven methods should be permitted and the Ministry of Health should retain its role as the sole supervisory body. Examples of already existing legal allowances made for podiatry and chiropractic were cited as examples of provisions that could be made for other NCM modalities once they were scientifically proven.

At the end of the day, the recommendations made by the committee were not adopted by the government and official regulation of NCM was not introduced, thereby perpetuating the current situation in which treatment of patients by non-MD NCM practitioners is against the law.

In 1995, the State Ombudsman's annual report dealt with the practice of NCM in Israel and the lack of implementation of the committee's recommendations. The situation in Israel was once more described as "far from satisfactory" because non-MD NCM practitioners were in effect neither supervised by professional bodies nor licensed by a legally recognized Israeli institution. Every practitioner was, in the words of the report, "a law unto himself."

The Israeli Medical Association (HARI) published its stand on the lack of regulation of NCM in Israel following publication of the State Ombudsman's report (no. 46) in November 1997. The response was formulated by the Israeli Medical Association's scientific committee. It stated that "there is no alternative medicine. There is one medicine alone that treats patients and this can be performed only by a licensed doctor. Obviously in the course of treatment a doctor is at liberty to choose the treatment most suited to his patient's condition." The clauses of the doctor's order (1976) are then repeated and the differences between conventional and alternative medicine reiterated. It is interesting to note that the Eilon Committee called NCM 'complementary medicine' whereas the medical association calls it 'alternative medicine' as a way of exoticizing and marginalizing it.

The basic argument presented by the Israeli Medical Association centered on the scientific status of conventional medicine as opposed to NCM modalities. "Alternative medicine" was described as a static entity based on a set of dogmas, whereas conventional medicine was represented as constantly reexamining itself by means of objective criteria. In weighing the basic principles of the freedom to seek treatment against the obligation to protect the public, HARI supports the latter and patients seeking NCM treatment are paternalistically described as being in a "vulnerable position" that necessitates the involvement and supervision of an attending doctor.

According to the outlook fostered by the Israeli Medical Association, NCM was divided into three main categories:

1. Practices that medicine recognizes as having a minimal benefit or does not totally object to such as acupuncture, chiropractic, and podiatry. These are deemed to have a theoretical basis and the practitioners undergo organized training of sorts.
2. Practices that medicine sees no clear benefit from such as homeopathy and herbs.
3. Practices that medicine clearly objects to (such as laying of hands) and views as charlatanism or witchcraft.

In the theoretical terms suggested in the previous chapter, this division matches the categories of selective integration (acupuncture, chiropractic, and podiatry), differentiation (homeopathy and herbs), and rejection (healing). Further on I will illustrate the processes by which NCM is acculturated and domesticated, as modalities such as homeopathy and herbalism move from the category of 'differentiation' into 'selective' integration and 'domestication.' The paradoxical stand adopted on herbalism and its categorization together with homeopathy as "having no particular benefit" is particularly interesting as articles (Perharic et al.,1993) have been published in medical journals as well as the popular press on the potential dangerous side effects of medicinal herbs. The solution ultimately recommended by HARI is that only MDs should be allowed to diagnose, treat, and prescribe. However, in the same manner that a doctor is assisted by paramedical professions such as nursing or physiotherapy, he or she may also be assisted by NCM practitioners of the first type (podiatrists, acupuncturists, and chiropractors), provided that they have undergone training and their work is carried out under medical supervision. Homeopathy and herbal remedies can be offered at the discretion of doctors who have some knowledge of these subjects.

The very conservative stand adopted by the Israeli Medical Association effectively curtailed any change in the status of NCM practitioners and reinstated the hegemony and dominance of the biomedical establishment in Israel. However, it is important to point out that even though not a single regulation or law was changed subsequent to the report's publication and the practice of NCM by non-MDs remained illegal and punishable, legal proceedings have rarely been initiated against NCM practitioners. In the absence of official regulation and supervision, a number of unofficial mechanisms have arisen that loosely direct the practice of NCM in Israel. These practices are particularly interesting as they represent a process of domestication that emerges on the grassroots level that is largely institutionalized but not legalized.

NCM Institutions in Israel

At present some 5,500 NCM practitioners are actively practicing in Israel and 450 teaching institutions exist (*Haaretz* 22.2.2002). However, only ten of these colleges offer extensive training courses that provide a diploma to graduates. It is important to note that these diplomas are not recognized by the Israeli Council for Higher Education but are usually granted in the framework of agreements between the colleges and similar institutions that exist either in China or the United States. This has not deterred Israelis from enrolling in the courses and it was estimated that by the end of 1999 some 110,000 Israelis had completed courses at the various NCM teaching institutions.

These schools have become agents of institutionalization as well as dissemination in the domestication of NCM in Israel. At present only two training institutions are affiliated with a recognized academic institution of learning. These are the School of Public Health at Bar-Ilan University, which offers a two-year program in NCM modalities that is open only to individuals who already have degrees in the health sciences (doctors, nurses, physical therapists), and the College of Management in Tel Aviv, which offers a recognized degree in biology along with an unrecognized one in NCM. Additional agents of institutionalization such as the Homeopathic Association for Doctors and Pharmacists in Israel have been established, although to date they have no formal standing concerning the government or supervisory status concerning practitioners.

In the absence of professional guidelines and state regulation, a mechanism of self-regulation has emerged, operated by self-appointed individuals or institutions. These institutions serve as cultural mediators, disseminating knowledge about the advantages and therapeutic possibilities of NCM to prospective patients, teaching therapeutic methods to students, and licensing them to practice with diplomas recognized neither by the Israeli Ministry of Health nor the Council for Higher Education. Parties involved in these colleges have also assumed the representation of the case of NCM to the legislative or medical authorities. In this manner the agenda has been set for the treatment and study of NCM in Israel by interested parties who also serve as cultural mediators. For this reason, I contend that the activities of such institutions (schools and clinics) are cardinal to the understanding of the growing popularity of NCM in Israel.

Clinics offering NCM therapies serve as major agents of domestication through consumption, institutionalization, and dissemination. Such clinics have become a popular venue through which the public consumes the services of NCM. Clinics also provide a meeting ground, a locus of interaction, for practitioners and patients. Two basic kinds of clinics exist in Israel: the multimodality NCM clinic adjacent to general hospitals and sick funds, and private clinics operated by a practitioner or a group of practitioners usually from home or in rooms that are part of a private medical complex. In the period between 1991 (the Committee's report) and 1998, the number of hospital-adjacent clinics grew from one to ten. Since Israel has twenty-two general hospitals this means that at least half of them operate some kind of NCM service. These clinics have been joined by NCM multimodality clinics operated by the large sick funds that are based on the same institutionalized pattern adopted by the hospital-affiliated clinics. Indeed all four Israeli HMOs operate NCM clinics and a total of fifty-seven such clinics exist (*Yediot* 19.10.2000). A large portion of NCM delivery in Israel is therefore administered through the hospital-adjacent or sick-fund-affiliated NCM clinics.

The NCM services provided by these institutions are not considered part of the "health basket" of covered services, but are usually partially subsidized in conjunction with the type of health coverage purchased by the member. The activities of these clinics are also prominently featured in the monthly news bulletins that the health funds send to their members. The clinics are controlled by MDs who see all patients first. After a preliminary examination by the clinic's MD who decides on a course of treatment, most patients are referred to a variety of therapies such as acupuncture, reflexology, shiatsu, chiropractic, biofeedback, hypnosis, homeopathy, and the Alexander technique. Grinstein et al. (2002) have pointed out that the establishment of these clinics by hospitals and HMOs is probably due to financial considerations in response to the authorization granted to the HMOs to market health services other than those included in the basket of public services. The HMOs correctly estimated the public's desire for NCM services, and provided these services to increase their own attractiveness and income. In this manner the public health system began to regard NCM as an important source of revenue and subsequently diminished its opposition to it. Undoubtedly, the fact that HMOs provide NCM services has served as an important legitimizing mechanism. In addition, it also domesticated NCM in the process.

Studying the encounter between conventional and NCM therapies within the framework of Israeli society provides a particularly interesting test case due to the fact that hardly any formal regulations are implemented by the Israeli State concerning the practice of NCM. At the informal level, although professional boards and registers have been established, they do not have a charter to enforce a code of ethics or conduct. For this reason, any regulatory practices are, in fact, self-regulatory and have evolved at the grass-roots level, probably reflecting the limitations perceived necessary by the NCM practitioners themselves. My contention is that these self-imposed limitations reflect a strategy for survival and expansion that take into account what the medical profession and the general public will or will not tolerate.

Methodological Considerations

This study sets out to explore the domestication of NCM in Israel through three major processes: dissemination (in the written press), institutionalization (in the NCM college and clinic), and consumption (in the NCM clinic). The focus on *processes* is in line with my analytical framework, which presupposes a dynamic *flow* of culture. The three processes studied were defined following a pilot study during which I attempted to map out the presence of NCM in the Israeli cultural field—collecting relevant media stories and visiting NCM institutions such as schools and clinics. Later on, during fieldwork, I focused on specific sites. The process of dissemination will be illustrated through an analysis of stories that appeared in the written press. Institutionalization will be described through well-known NCM colleges; and consumption is analyzed by examining one of the established clinics, its practitioners, and its patients. Selecting one locus for observation and analysis reflected the ethnographic necessity of defining the field's boundaries. The generalizability of each of these 'cases' is discussed in the beginning of each chapter.

There is, of course, a strong linkage among the three processes that I describe, and the selection of ethnographic loci represents that

Setting the Scene

linkage. The clinic chosen for observation is molded after a hospital unit, with practitioners working at the clinic (many of them MDs) also serving on the faculties of various NCM colleges. Students at these colleges would also come and observe at the clinic and perform supervised practical work there. NCM stories in the written press are often based on interviews given by practitioners working at various clinics. The ethnography combines all three basic sources of qualitative data gathering—observation, textual analysis, and interviews (Denzin, 1978). In addition, a questionnaire based on interviews conducted with patients attending the clinic was compiled and administered to some three hundred patients at the clinic to examine their attitudes and beliefs on a number of issues. A control group of the same size as the experimental group was also similarly studied. In order to try and match the medical problems characteristic of patients attending the NCM clinic, the patients constituting the control group were recruited from an orthopedic and an allergy outpatient clinic. A quantitative analysis of data derived from the questionnaires is presented in the chapter on the patients.

Research at the clinic was conducted during a period of five years, from 1992 to 1997. During this time I observed the clinic's public and backstage domains and interviewed patients before and after treatment, sometimes encountering the same patient three or four times. I maintained contact with some of the practitioners working at the clinic, again conducting ongoing conversations over a period of months, sometimes years. In this manner issues could be worked out, understood, and questions and thoughts shared. I also attended lectures given by the practitioners at different forums outside of, as well as within, the hospital framework; I was present at seminars held by the clinic and, during the last two years of fieldwork, was also admitted to the monthly staff meetings. During the period of observation, changes occurred at the clinic—it moved into new quarters, practitioners came and went—although a hard core remained, and competing institutions were established.

A similar multifaceted approach has been adopted by Lupton (1994) in her study of medicine as a cultural phenomenon. Lupton claimed that

> There is much to be gained from an eclectic perspective which approaches the same research problem from different theoretical and methodological angles... the potential exists for the

different theoretical approaches and research methodologies to incorporate elements from each other to meet their own deficiencies, and perhaps, in the process, to weaken the boundaries that tend rather artificially to separate them (1994: 19).

In the framework of this study, for example, information elicited through observation of case presentations at staff meetings could not have been obtained by means of a questionnaire. Conversely, the waiting area situation often did not provide the privacy necessary for conducting interviews with patients, and therefore a self-reporting questionnaire was considered a more suitable tool for learning about patients' expectations, beliefs, and health problems. I believe that my use of various research methods, qualitative as well as quantitative, contributed to understanding the heterogeneity, cultural complexity, and richness of NCM.

I have followed Gubrium's (1988) lead in framing my ethnography around structures that mediate between participants and discourses. Such structures are loosely defined as frames that influence the construction of attitudes and practices among people. These structures can be geographically localized and physically bounded, as in the case of 'places' such as the clinic or the college. However, they can also be geographically dispersed and unbound by place—as in the case of the media. The clinic, the college, and the media are grouped together under the term "structures" since all of them have a major role in the construction of attitudes regarding NCM. My analysis focuses on the structures that facilitate and constrain the practice of NCM; the people, the actors in the field, are examined through their reactions to and participation in these structures. My argument is that these structures are dynamic loci of negotiation between the conventional and the alternative.

Chapter 3

Negotiation: The NCM Clinic

Although the NCM clinic I studied was loosely affiliated with a hospital, there was in fact little cooperation in the form of patient referral or joint consultation. The fact that the clinic was adjacent to the hospital, however, established a sense of respectability, security, and legitimacy for many patients. In interviews conducted with the clinic's patients many stated that the fact that the clinic was "part of a hospital" afforded a sense of security as to the nature and quality of care that they expected to receive. The symbolic patronage of the hospital was perceived, in other words, as a reassuring sign of acculturation. It definitely served to differentiate the complementary clinic from practitioners who operated from private clinics or from their homes. A similar observation was made by Schneirov and Gezcik (2002) in a study conducted at an NCM clinic located in an urban hospital in the United States.

The multitherapy, multipractitioner, hospital-affiliated clinic has gained much popularity in the Israeli context. By 1999, ten of the twenty-two general hospitals in Israel had NCM clinics associated with them, all of which operated in a similar method to the one described in this study. Moreover, the major health funds have established NCM clinics offering services to their members at a reduced price. In 2000, fifty-seven of these clinics existed and operated in the same manner as the hospital-adjacent clinics. The clinic under study can therefore be viewed as representative of this mode of NCM treatment delivered in Israel. Moreover, the chapter on patients shows that those who have used NCM prefer biomedical supervision, irrespective

---

Some details in the case studies have been changed to protect the identity of the patients. Pseudonyms are used throughout this chapter.

of the venue where treatment was received. Obviously, NCM treatments are also administered by individual practitioners operating out of private rooms or their homes. This cannot, however, be viewed as "private" practice of NCM in contrast to the clinic practices as the services provided by the clinics are indeed "private" and paid for out-of-pocket. Due to the legal situation of NCM in Israel, described in the previous chapter, it is difficult to estimate the number of unaffiliated practitioners and the scope of their practices. One can also expect great variance in the practices of unaffiliated NCM practitioners as a result of the lack of uniformity in training. Although these practitioners provide a potentially interesting field for further study, it is my contention that the NCM multimodality clinic in Israel constitutes a large part of NCM practice and that processes observed at these clinics are molding the relationship between conventional and nonconventional medicine in Israel. Indeed these clinics provide a cultural meeting place for the negotiation of the future status and character of NCM.

The Clinic and Its Boundaries

The clinic can be perceived as situated within a physical as well as a symbolic setting. The boundaries of both settings were constantly being negotiated as the clinic established its existence. The clinic was opened in the early 1990s and was one of the first of its kind in Israel. It was situated on the grounds of a large general hospital in the center of the country. In the first years it was not allotted its own exclusive area in the hospital, but shared rooms with a modern outpatient unit that was situated close to the hospital's main entrance. For this reason the decor was not something that the clinic controlled. The wall-to-wall carpeting, matte black formica and chrome tables, and low, dark upholstered chairs, luxurious by general hospital standards, gave the area a dignified appearance. On the inside wall facing the glass double doors through which one entered was a transparent Plexiglass plaque listing all the different treatments available. To the left of the entrance was the secretaries' post—a large, low L-shaped desk with two computers.

A little before 3 P.M.—on days when the clinic operated in the afternoon—Barbara, the secretary, picked up a box containing small, self-adhesive signs and made her way along the maroon-carpeted floor.

The clinic, which had functioned as an outpatient unit during the morning hours, was now changing its designation and becoming the NCM clinic. With a bit of adhesive tape, the room marked Endocrinology was now labeled Acupuncture, Cardiology became Reflexology, and so on. The consulting rooms, designed to meet traditional medical needs, were furnished with a desk, a large chair for the physician, two chairs on the opposite side for the patient and his or her companion, and an examination couch. The rooms also often contained sophisticated machinery, which of course had no bearing on the NCM consultation, but was nevertheless present and constructed a symbolic space of technological-medical reality. This technological "decor," a residual of what had occurred in these rooms during the morning, was obsolete in the afternoon; nevertheless, its presence could not be ignored.

The fact that the clinic was situated on the grounds of a large general hospital and called "Secomed adjacent to Farmer's General Hospital" (names are fictive) led many patients to believe that the NCM clinic was in fact an integral unit of the hospital. Patients would often arrive thinking that the clinic constituted part of the services to which a sick-fund patient was entitled free of charge and were surprised to hear that a considerable fee (between $50 and $60 for the first consultation depending on the period) was charged. On learning that the service was not free, these patients would usually decide to forgo their appointment and leave the clinic.

When the clinic moved to its own exclusive quarters—a renovated hangar near the new wing that it had formerly occupied—the decor, while not as plush as before, remained office-like.[1] The floors were covered with a light blue-gray, wall-to-wall carpet, and the chairs in the waiting area were also upholstered in a light fabric. The consulting rooms were furnished with a desk, two chairs, and an examination couch. Toward the back of the unit was a large area— too small to be called a hall—in which meetings and workshops were held. It is noteworthy that even after the clinic received its own quarters, the decor was not contrived to reflect an experience of "otherness" or of stepping out of day-to-day experience. There was no Chinese calligraphy or art on the walls, no therapeutic residue such as bottles, needles, or dried herbs, and no incense, dimmed lights, or background "mood" music.

The clinic was constantly attempting to extend its symbolic boundaries in a number of ways:

1. **Research.** An attempt was made to create interest in joint research projects with various departments at the hospital. This was problematic due to the difficulty of obtaining funding for research in NCM and probably also the reluctance of established departments to finance this type of research. One of the main problems of NCM vis-à-vis conventional medicine was the demand to provide scientific proof according to accepted experimental protocol. The clinic's attempts to initiate research projects were usually met with interest, but failed to garner funding.

2. **Consultation.** The clinic was eager to offer its services within the hospital wards, thereby extending its boundaries from physical affiliation to clinical involvement. This was not well received. The two cases in which the clinic's services were called on that I know of were: (1) a child with severe hepatitis who was not responding to conventional treatment. The NCM clinic was asked to offer a remedy. The case was so acute that the NCM physician consulted (informally) commented with disdain that at that stage "even putting a dove on the child's belly" (a practice common in folk healing) would do as much good; (2) a female teenager with acute, recurrent abdominal pain of psychosomatic origin. In this case, an MD who specialized in internal medicine treated the patient in the emergency department with NCM methods, apparently with success.

3. **Workshops, Seminars, and Conferences.** The clinic was constantly arranging events of this type to which hospital staff, NCM practitioners working at the clinic as well as those unaffiliated with it, certain patients, staff at other hospitals, and media representatives would all be invited. These events were often poorly (almost embarrassingly so) attended. They were usually held in the hospital auditorium and consisted of short speeches made by a representative of the hospital's administrative staff, the MD in charge of the clinic, and case presentations in which one or two patients would describe their medical problem and then a clinic-affiliated MD would rephrase the problem and describe the treatment and its outcome. The audience was invited to participate and ask questions. At one such gathering there was also an artistic program in which a Chinese therapist who practiced a kind of dance therapy demonstrated his art to

the sound of Oriental-type gong music. The audience was told that he would be affiliated with the clinic pending his return from a visit home to China. As far as I know he never returned. His picture did, however, appear in the local newspapers together with a report on the conference. The spokesperson of another large general hospital commented to me that in her opinion the NCM clinic had invited "all the wrong people." Understanding that the purpose of these functions was to a large extent PR, inviting people who "are already convinced" was, in her opinion "a waste of time." The question as to whether the unconvinced had the time or the inclination to attend such functions, either in the middle of a working day or after work hours, remains unanswered.

4. **The Media.** The media served as a powerful vehicle for creating public awareness of the clinic's existence and the therapeutic options it had to offer. The first-person narrative accounts featured in many articles were viewed in the clinic as creating a kind of therapeutic community, which drew prospective patients to the realm of NCM through identification.

Through these efforts, the clinic was determined to capture more "symbolic space" for itself among professionals and the lay public alike.

How the Clinic Worked

First Contact

Visits to the clinic were by appointment only. On the first visit, prior to commencing treatment, the patient was seen by an MD. This was to diagnose the patient's condition in conventional terms, discover what tests and treatments had been used, and decide which alternative therapy would most likely be beneficial for that particular patient. The sorting MD assumed ultimate therapeutic responsibility for the patient, supervising progress and providing medico-legal cover for the treatments administered by non-MD therapists. The sorting MD was expected to go through patients' files at regular intervals and contact those who had discontinued treatment prematurely. If a patient had persevered with treatment that had not been successful, the MD would refer the patient to a different therapy. During the initial consultation, the sorting MD would examine the patient, take down the medical history, and explain the various options available and also why a particular method had been chosen. The MD would try to establish a therapeutic relationship with the patient, letting him or her participate in making a joint decision on the nature of treatment. Most patients were satisfied with the attention they received at the sorting interview. Others, however, were not. The therapeutic alliance, verbally cemented in terms such as "let's try this," "let's see what this does for you," or "what would you say to . . ." confused them and made them feel that they were not getting their money's worth. They had come for a solution, were paying good money for it, and could not cope with tentativeness. Indeed, several patients did not show up for treatment subsequent to the sorting consultation. This was a source of bewilderment for practitioners at the clinic, who, in line with clinic policy, saw the sorting consultation as a necessary first step in a long process. It was assumed that these patients had perhaps used the clinic's services in order to ascertain what sort of treatment best suited their complaint and then sought treatment elsewhere. Although data is not available on this issue, a man whose daughter had successfully been treated at the clinic provided proof for this assumption. He consulted with the sorting doctor for his complaint. When shiatsu was suggested as a therapeutic option, the man decided to be treated by his wife who had just completed a course on the subject.

The sorting doctor also assumed responsibility toward all practitioners at the clinic for fair distribution of cases (the practitioners were remunerated on a per-case basis). This obviously placed the doctor in a political position. A conversation between the MD in charge of the clinic and a new sorting doctor (a specialist in pediatrics) illustrates this point. The sorting doctor was showing the MD in charge a list of patients he had seen that afternoon. "Look how neatly it worked out today," he said, "two for reflexology, one for medicinal herbs, two for nutrition. . . ." "How old was the child you referred to medicinal herbs?" the chief cut him short. "Twelve," he responded. "Well, that's probably all right then; children younger than that usually find the herbal potions too bitter and don't persevere." Decisions about the type of treatment to be preferred therefore did not stem from potential therapeutic benefit alone, but from an overall impression of the patient as well as the structural needs of the clinic to provide work for the practitioners associated with it.

Treatment and Perseverance

Once the patient had consulted the sorting doctor, the next step was an appointment with the designated practitioner. This usually did not happen on the same day and the patient would often have to wait a week or even two for an appointment. One patient told me she was very disgruntled because she had had two appointments at which forms had been filled in and she had already paid about $60 yet had not actually been treated. This was aggravated by the fact that the therapist had arrived late for the appointment. The patient's complaint was not dealt with by the secretary beyond the perfunctory remark, "I'm very sorry but there's nothing we can do about it," and the doctor in charge subsequently received a letter of complaint. The therapist was instructed to give the patient one free treatment.

The secretaries, whose desk was situated at the entrance to the clinic, scheduled appointments and received payments and therefore often served as targets for dissatisfaction or, conversely, compliments. Patients were well aware that they were paying private fees and subsequently demanded appropriate treatment. Treatments administered at the clinic (for an annotated list, see the Appendix) can be divided into two main groups: repetitive and nonrepetitive. Repetitive treatments were administered once or twice a week and usually included manual therapies such as shiatsu, reflexology, or acupuncture, or types of exercise such as the Paula technique, the Alexander technique, or Feldenkreis exercising. A course of about twelve treatments was recommended before improvement could be noticed. Patients often discontinued the prescribed course of treatment before it had been completed. This was a continuous source of frustration for the therapists who felt that the patient had not given the method a fair chance to prove itself. The nonrepetitive treatments, such as homeopathy, herbalism, Chinese medicine, or dietary control presented an entirely different set of problems. Improvement in health following homeopathic treatment or dietary monitoring was sometimes only experienced after a month or six weeks. In the interim patients tended to "get lost." Often improvement was gradual and then it was not attributed to the treatment, or if the condition was temporarily aggravated—a good sign, in homeopathic treatment—patients would tend to fall back on conventional means. Remedying this situation was difficult. Patients were encouraged to contact the practitioner with any problem or question that might arise during this period, and if a patient did not maintain contact with the clinic after the first consultation, practitioners were required to make contact and inquire what had happened.

The topic of perseverance was much discussed and various ideas on achieving compliance were always being entertained. One of the explanations for low compliance, expressed by prematurely severing the therapeutic relationship, was attributed to patients' high expectations from treatment. To remedy this situation, practitioners were urged to converse with patients during treatments and impress upon them that improvement would be gradual. "Get their expectations down," they were told time and again. One attempt to ascertain that a patient would indeed complete the full course of treatment prescribed was to demand advance payment for the entire series. Patients did not usually view this request favorably, preferring to see if there was any improvement and then make the decision whether or not to continue. Tension existed at times between the secretaries and management about advance payment. Secretaries reported problems on this issue and the management insisted that greater efforts must be made. The attempt to ask people who called up to make their first appointment for their credit card number in order to ensure that the appointment was kept was unsuccessful too; it was also unpopular with the secretaries, who claimed that it caused unpleasantness and elicited antagonism.

Leaving the Clinic

Obviously the best reason for discontinuing treatment was due to cure or alleviation of symptoms. This was, however, difficult to measure as complaints were often of a subjective nature. Some patients, whose symptoms had been relieved, returned for treatment after a period of time due to recurrence of the original health problem or something new cropping up. In these cases the patient would not undergo the entire sorting process from the beginning, but would make an appointment with a specific practitioner.

Patients often severed treatment because they felt that they had not been cured. In these cases, clinic staff often believed that the patients had given neither the clinic nor the method a fair chance, and that contact had been prematurely ended. From the clinic's point of view, when a patient was not experiencing improvement, that patient should return to the sorting doctor for further consultation and a joint decision would be made as to which other method could be tried. Although this situation was the "ideal situation" from the clinic's point of view, patients usually did not persevere that long with what they perceived as "unsuccessful (and costly) treatment." Dissatisfied patients were indeed a bad advertisement for the clinic and patients who had discontinued treatment, or canceled appointments without rescheduling, were contacted either by the sorting MD or the therapist who had administered treatment in order to tactfully inquire "how they were feeling."

The Staff

The clinic staff was composed of a fairly stable core of practitioners—MDs and non-MDs. Apart from the MD in charge of the clinic, the other affiliates maintained a part-time relationship, working at the clinic one or two full or half days a week. Other practitioners, who came and went in the course of time during which I observed the clinic, usually became affiliated with similar institutes. The MDs were dominant in running the clinic and the fact that an MD always occupied the position of the sorting doctor enhanced their already powerful position in setting the clinic's agenda. At staff meetings MDs were much more likely to attend than non-MDs, probably because the MDs were much more involved in clinic politics. In any event, involvement—whether stable and long term or short term and erratic—was always on a part-time basis. Affiliation with the clinic was considered desirable from the point of view of the interprofessional pecking order. Non-MD practitioners drew professional legitimacy from being affiliated with a "hospital" clinic, as did the MDs. There were some claims that practitioners took advantage of their affiliation with the clinic to transfer patients from the clinic to their private practices. There was some truth to these charges, although nothing operative was (or could be) done to prevent this practice.

Three secretaries were employed by the clinic, all on a part-time basis. In principle the phones were answered throughout the day, but the main activity was usually during the afternoon hours when most practitioners preferred to work. Their responsibilities included directing patients to the correct consulting room, filling in forms, distributing files, making repeat appointments, taking payment, and dealing with telephone inquiries and appointments. Despite this pressure, they knew many patients by name and their friendly attitude was often commented on.

Uniforms

In the beginning, when the clinic was established, all staff members were formally required to wear the clinic's shirt. This shirt was short-sleeved and round-necked, with pop-studs down the front, and made of polyester. It was beige with green trimming and had the clinic insignia—a leaf held between thumb and forefinger—printed on the front. The style was that of the traditional, hospital-like white shirt donned by medical staff. A secretary had selected the color. When I asked her why she had selected that particular color, she said that it was just about the only one left. "Doctors wear white, so that's out of the question—we're not even allowed to use that color; green is the color of operating theater clothing; the patients' pajamas are apricot or light blue; dark blue is the color manual workers wear—so there wasn't much of a choice." The uniform shirt, however, was not popular. The women, secretaries and therapists, all complained that it was boxy and unflattering. As a compromise, some wore it open over their clothes. Aside from the doctor in charge of the clinic, I never saw the shirt worn by a male therapist—MDs and non-MDs alike. Therapists opted to forgo the use of "professional" garb altogether, preferring their own clothing. The MDs were usually neatly attired in button-down shirts and the other therapists adopted an "earthy," casual type of appearance and wore large T-shirts and sandals. MDs were requested not to wear their white hospital tops while working at the clinic so that they would not create the impression that they were under hospital auspices. This rule was usually observed, with the exception of one MD who came over from one of the hospital wards—thus introducing another type of "day residue" into the scene. As a researcher studying the clinic and approaching patients for interviews, I was also awarded a beige shirt, which I did not wear. The shirt, unpopular from the start, was very quickly discarded and therapists would just wear their ordinary day-to-day apparel.

The attempt to enforce uniformity through dress is one aspect of the desire to present a homogeneous front, modeled on the hospital ward or clinic. The unpopularity of the beige shirt is especially noteworthy when juxtaposed with the universal adoption of a white or green uniform by all staff in the conventional clinic or hospital setting, from the cleaning lady to the chief of surgery. This could perhaps indicate rejection of symbolic uniformity in the NCM clinic.

Moreover, the fact that both MDs and non-MDs practiced the same type of NCM did not serve as a flattening mechanism. In interviews that

I conducted with the MD practitioners, there was almost uniform agreement that they were "first a doctor and then a homeopath," or whatever other therapy they happened to practice. In the case of the establishment of professional associations, for example, there was one association solely for homeopathic doctors that barred entrance to all other non-MD homeopaths, irrespective of the place or nature of their training. There are a number of institutions and teachers of homeopathy around the world that are very highly thought of. The fact that a non-MD might have studied at one of these institutions would not admit him or her into the association of MD homeopaths. Conversely, the nature or quality of the homeopathic training of the MDs was not an issue that would bar, or facilitate, entry into the association.

Non-MD practitioners were well aware of the higher status of MDs. Throughout my observations, the issue of registration and licensing occupied therapists, and reports on progress made or discussions held with Health Ministry functionaries were discussed at many of the meetings. It is interesting to note that a variety of sources, affiliated with the clinic or the colleges, repeatedly informed me that the matter of licensing, regulation, and registration was "on the brink of being settled" and that "too much discussion or an unnecessary word could ruin the entire process." To date, no official legislation has been formulated or implemented. The position assumed by the Israeli Medical Association is extremely conservative, reserving the hegemony of the conventional medical establishment in defining, diagnosing, and treating illness. The fact that this stand might be legally enforced was worrisome for non-MD practitioners. At one meeting a non-MD homeopath urged the MD reporting on "progress" made at one such meeting with Health Ministry officials that the MDs recognize their "responsibility towards the non-MD practitioners who are numerous and sometimes well established professionally."

The following section describes staff meetings held at the clinic. In the last year of my research I was able to attend eight staff meetings, whose focal point was a case presented for discussion. This allowed me to examine one of the innermost circles of discourse on NCM that was being conducted by the professional community among and for itself.

The Staff Meeting

Staff meetings, which were held in the evening on a monthly basis, were sporadically attended by practitioners working at the clinic. Two

MD's, Dr. Nadler, who had founded the clinic and acted as its coordinator, and Dr. Binnaker were always present. Sometimes the sorting doctors such as Dr. Beauchamps, Dr. Kipp, or Dr. Ramah were present, although not very often. The rest of the practitioners, who were not MDs, attended more or less at whim and attendance was usually between ten and fifteen practitioners.

The meetings were presided over by Dr. Nadler, who would open with an administrative survey that generally covered such subjects as the clinic's financial situation, names of institutions that had signed agreements with the clinic (thus entitling their members to a preferential fee), and ways to increase the volume of patients visiting the clinic and retain those who had commenced treatment. The latter issue was a major cause of concern since patients who severed their relationship with the clinic before being cured were a bad advertisement and a source of frustration for practitioners. Numerous attempts were made to devise methods of ascertaining that a patient persevered for the duration of a prescribed course of treatment. For example, practitioners administering manual therapies were instructed to talk to the patients during the therapeutic session (which lasted for about half an hour) and constantly emphasize the point that improvement would be gradual. Practitioners such as homeopaths or nutritionists were asked to telephone patients at home to find out how they were feeling and offer support, advice, and sympathy. Moreover, the sorting doctors, who assumed medical responsibility for the patient and supervised the treatments administered by non-MDs, were supplied with computer printouts of patients who had ended contact with the clinic. The doctors were required to telephone these people and find out the reason for the premature termination of the therapeutic relationship. In reality, it was difficult to implement this demand because it was time-consuming, a list of patients quickly formed, and a number of calls were necessary before the patient was actually reached. For this reason, adherence to this practice soon petered out. All practitioners were expected, however, to be available for patients to contact between treatments.

After administrative topics had been dealt with, the meeting moved on to its academic focus—the case presentation. A case chosen by the unit responsible for the particular meeting was written up and a typed version distributed to all present. The practitioner presenting the case then led the discussion and answered questions on the treatment administered and its outcome.

Case Presentations

The first case was presented by an MD trained as a homeopath, who was at the time also acting as a sorting doctor. The case was in the format of any conventional medical write-up, with allowances made for the fact that not all those reading the document had the medical knowledge necessary to understand it and therefore qualifying remarks were added for the benefit of the non-MD practitioners, who constituted the majority of participants in the discussion. The case description was divided into subsections: chief complaint; examinations and tests performed; medical history. The next section of the case dealt with the patient's medical condition on examination and the type of treatment chosen for her.

Case 1—A Swallowing Disorder

The patient, Betty, a forty-year-old married mother of four who worked as a secretary, complained of dysphagia—a swallowing disorder, as the non-MDs were informed in brackets. The problem apparently arose five months prior to the present consultation when the woman had been hospitalized following acute inflammation of the gall bladder. In the course of hospitalization, insertion of a gastric tube was required and since then she has complained of difficulty swallowing, especially solids, the sensation of a lump in her throat, and heartburn. The patient reported a weight loss of 20-odd kg that she attributed to her complaint as well as to some sort of diet (no details were given in the case history).

The examinations were described in detail, once again with bracketed explanations for the benefit of non-MDs. Treatment administered with Adalat (Nifedipine—a drug that blocks calcium and relaxes the smooth muscle) was mentioned. Details of all other medications taken were also given, sometimes with the exact dosage. For example, stomach acidity was treated with Zantac (Ranitidine) 150 mg twice daily. In general, the examinations and tests did not detect any physiological basis for the complaint. These details were somewhat superfluous considering the professional audience, which they were aimed at. The non-MD practitioners were unable to ask informed questions concerning the tests, their outcome, medication, and dosage. Furthermore, they were unable to suggest additional testing or recommend other medication.

The psychological aspects of stress and anxiety were then discussed as part of the patient's medical history. Betty was reported as describing herself as always being "restless" with no apparent reason. She could not single out any stressful event or particular anxiety that might have occurred at the time her complaint emerged. Moreover, the patient did not seem to connect her swallowing problem with her general anxiety. It is interesting to note that although the doctor presenting the case conceded that the complaint might be connected to psychological stress, she did not point to the emergency hospitalization and surgery as possible stress factors, which could have triggered the problem in the first place.

The report goes on to describe in detail what the MD saw as excessive use of tranquilizers and sleeping pills. At the time of her initial consultation at the clinic, practitioners were informed, Betty was taking Xanax (Alprazolan) prescribed by her family physician who also had the impression that stress was at the source of her problem. Although this medication led to neither physical nor psychological improvement, the patient continued taking it. In addition, she reported sleeping disturbances, which were treated with Vaben (Oxazepam), Lorivan (Lorazepan), and lately Bondormin (Brotizolam) on a regular basis. At the time of the consultation the patient was seeing a psychiatrist who was treating her with Melodil (maprotiline, an antianxiety and antidepressant agent) together with psychotherapy. She reported mediocre to slight improvement.

After describing the patient's medical background, the presenting MD evaluated the patient's present condition in the following manner:

> Physical examination was without findings. I got the impression that the patient was under considerable stress, but did not succeed in focusing on the problem or the sense of stress, which the patient talked about. I did not get the impression that the patient was depressed or suffering from any other psychiatric disorder. It is my feeling that it is most likely that the physical complaints stem from the patient's sense of stress together with another important element of treatment, excessive use of sedatives with a suspicion of addiction.

The diagnosis therefore placed the complaint in the realm of the psychosomatic and also indirectly blamed the treatment given by conventional medicine for aggravating the problem.

The choice of treatment for the patient was shiatsu due to the pronounced element of stress and the impression that she needed therapy through touch. Nutrition therapy was recommended together with the shiatsu, but the patient was unwilling to comply because she had already been treated by a nutritionist at her sick fund. The use of the Paula technique was rejected because the impression was that the patient would not be able to comply with the exercise regime. Homeopathy was not recommended at this primary stage because it was felt that the patient needed a repetitive framework, at least once a week, due to the characteristics of dependence mentioned. The patient was not interested in reflexology as a result of past experience with the method. The patient duly commenced shiatsu treatment with Donna (a practitioner at the clinic). After two treatments, and following a conversation between the reporting physician and Donna, the patient was referred to Dr. Binnaker for concomitant treatment with medicinal herbs in order to gradually wean her from the sleep-inducing sedatives through the introduction of a "natural substitute" (inverted quotation marks in the original). Up to this point, the patient had had nine shiatsu treatments. She reported a sense of relaxation and an alleviation of symptoms, which lasted for about two days after the treatment and then returned. She did not persevere with the herbs.

At present, the report continued, the patient had stopped shiatsu treatment. Her complaints had generally been relieved to a moderate degree. They still continued to bother her, though not on a daily basis. The nature of the complaint had also changed somewhat: the patient experienced the sensation that "something is stuck in her throat," a sensation relieved by eating. End of case report.

This case is an epitome of the "problem patient" who tends to frustrate the medical profession. Her complaint is of a psychosomatic nature, which the extensive use of both conventional and nonconventional methods has not cured. Once a complaint is phrased, or diagnosed, as nonphysiological, cure can only be achieved through the patient's becoming aware of the psychological etiology of the complaint. The ensuing discussion of the case was conducted entirely in the realm of psychosomatic medicine and although the objective of the discussion was to try and solve the patient's problem, the case actually served as an outlet for the practitioners' frustration at the type of patient who did not get well because he or she "resisted" treatment. To make things worse, this patient could not be labeled noncompliant. She had in fact undergone nine treatments in shiatsu.

The discussion of the case probed into possible secondary gains attached to the woman's illnesses, past and present, and it was also suggested that her complaints might have been the result of the trauma of hospitalization, particularly the insertion of a gastric tube. Dr. Binnaker comically referred to the discomfort of gastric intubation, reminiscing: "once upon a time when we were 'bad' [meaning conventional—J. F.] doctors working in the emergency ward we used stomach intubation to 'teach patients a lesson,' like when a woman would turn up at the ward and say 'I took an overdose.'" The recourse to "humor" to describe and then dissociate oneself from an uncomfortable, invasive procedure is noteworthy.

It is also interesting that the possibility of hospital-induced trauma was not included in the write-up. However, when this point was raised at the meeting, the reporting MD immediately agreed that this was a plausible explanation. This could possibly be due to the fact that the MD did not want to take a stand in blaming conventional medical treatment—in any case, not in a written document. Responsibility for lack of progress, however, was entirely the patient's. This was either because the patient was on a "low plane of self-consciousness" or "afraid to get well." "What should we do with that kind of patient," despaired Dr. Binnaker, "except tell her that she needs a minimum of twenty treatments and then she will relax and not be afraid that she will suddenly go and get herself well."

Dr. Diamond wondered out loud what benefit such a patient could gain from psychiatric treatment as she (in his words) "was not on a very high level of self-consciousness on one hand, while producing a high level of somatization on the other." "I'll tell you what she talks about," said Dr. Binnaker, "she talks about the fact that she can't swallow. And if there just might be a spark of revelation, if she just might touch on something real, or the psychiatrist might broach a matter, she will say 'Yes ... but my throat. ...'"

Dr. Greer, an MD practicing homeopathy, who was present at the particular meeting, could sympathize with the general notion of the patient who refuses to get well by contributing an anecdote from her own practice. Greer told the story of Nell, whose husband she had cured of asthma. The homeopathic consultation with Nell lasted for an hour and a half, at the end of which Dr. Greer gave her one capsule. "One capsule!" Nell exclaimed, " One capsule! Is that all you can give me? I have been suffering from this pain for fifteen years and what you give me is one capsule!" Nell did not return for follow-up treatment. Greer explained that it is difficult for the patient to part with her pain. The pain is very much hers, it belongs to her, it is part of her being.

A theme that was brought up for discussion following the case study and Dr. Greer's anecdote was whether it was worthwhile to refer the hysterical, somatic type of patient to conventional diagnostic tests in order to prove to the individual that "nothing is wrong physically." This was an interesting conjecture because it reified the connection between pathological abnormality and symptoms, a connection foreign to the holistic body-mind ideology of NCM. Reification of pathological etiology and recognition of a split between body and mind leads to an additional division, the subjective as opposed to the objective, with the latter being granted greater legitimacy than the former. Strictly speaking, this division is contrary to the ideology of NCM, which emphasizes a subjective, holistic, patient-centered worldview. The subjective definition of symptoms was addressed by a chiropractor present, who said that the body had a language of its own with which the therapist should go along. He provided the example of a ballet dancer he was treating. Although no physiological evidence was observable, the dancer complained of pain and so the chiropractor "treated her pain."

Ultimately, no decision was reached on the subject. It is important to note, however, that the entire discussion was conducted in the terminology and tradition of conventional medicine. Recourse to the objectivity of laboratory tests as a therapeutic means was discussed as part of the process of proving to a patient that "nothing is wrong" with him or her and thereby justifying the move into the realm of psychosomatic and subjective complaints. An alternative discourse of diagnosis and healing did not emerge in the discussion at the staff meeting. The perspective adopted could have just as well been discussed in a forum of conventional medicine. The manner in which the discussion was conducted—moving from the psychological to the physical—did not seem to embody an "alternative view" of the problem, but rather a repetition of the conventional view within a different setting.

In the course of this discussion a non-MD practitioner of traditional Chinese medicine addressed Dr. Nadler, an MD who practiced acupuncture. "You know," she said, "Chinese medicine has a name for such a condition. It is a condition characteristic of middle-aged women and is called the "plum-stuck-in-the-throat" syndrome. Chinese medicine also has a specific therapy for this syndrome." "You're quite right! Very good, very good indeed!" exclaimed Nadler, happy at her display of professional prowess. The forum present was not, however, offered an explanation of the syndrome and its cure in the terms of Chinese medicine. This alternative language was neither made common nor afforded attention. This might be because, at that particular meeting, the four MDs (herbalist, naturopath, homeopath, and acupuncturist) and the non-MD practitioners were not versed, nor perhaps even interested in, traditional Chinese medicine. This once again serves to prove that conventional medicine dominated the meeting as the only common frame of reference.

Case 2 — A Homeopathic Interview

The next case study, brought up for discussion at another staff meeting, generated far less discussion than Betty's dysphagia, probably because it described successful treatment and a compliant patient. Two background factors should be noted. First, this case study was written up and presented to the meeting by a practitioner who had no formal, conventional medical training; and second, the homeopathic diagnosis called attention to experiential and behavioral factors in addition to physical aspects. For this reason, this case was somewhat different from the one presented earlier. The forum's overall reaction, however, was similar.

The case concerned a woman who had been diagnosed as suffering from Chronic Fatigue Syndrome (CFS). Before the presentation of the case by Justine, a non-MD homeopath, Dr. Binnaker gave a clinical update on CFS and discussed the difficulty in diagnosing the syndrome, thereby framing the case in the terminology of conventional medicine. The update provided a historical and scientific review of the syndrome and referred to an article published in *The Lancet* (a prestigious medical journal). One of the problems described in Dr. Binnaker's review was the general hesitance in deciding whether to label the presenting set of symptoms as CFS. Dr. Binnaker pointed out that sometimes the diagnosis was made when the syndrome was, in fact, absent. On the other hand, because antibodies could appear some time after the patient has suffered symptoms, there were cases in which the syndrome was present but went undiagnosed. This was an interesting point as it illustrated the importance of the conventional diagnostic label in the construction of illness.

This talk provided a conventional medical framework for the homeopath's presentation. However, it was also somewhat irrelevant since the homeopathic paradigm does not take the actual sickness into account, but concentrates more on the patient's specific symptoms as the basis for prescribing a remedy. Once again the alternative paradigm was not allowed to provide the framework for discussion and was replaced by the general paradigm of conventional medicine. Another potential conflict could emerge from the "medical fact" that a CFS patient might not have been "really" sick in the first place, rendering the cure as "non-cure."

Lily, a forty-year-old married woman, mother of two children aged seventeen and nineteen, first visited the clinic in February 1995 because of CFS that had been diagnosed one year earlier. It all had started, the homeopath recounted, three years ago as flu and nausea. Lily used to wake up every morning with terrible nausea, fatigue, and general weakness; severe loss of appetite; and blurring of vision. The patient underwent a long series of tests and examinations, which were normal. The possibility was raised that she was suffering from the Epstein-Barr virus. At the time she was given Prozac and felt her usual self within three weeks. However, every subsequent illness that entailed treatment with antibiotics led to a new recurrence. She suffered repeatedly from bronchitis. For the past two years she had been treated by reflexology. Up to now she had had thirty-six reflexology treatments and three months ago she gradually started to decrease the dosage of Prozac. She still takes the drug every day, but in a lower dosage. There was some improvement with reflexology, but she still felt weak and exhausted, tired, impatient, and had no appetite. An "attack" always started with a decrease in appetite. In bad periods she slept heavily. Sleep was unpleasant; she dreamt that she was sinking into some place and had nightmares. The homeopath then moved on to describe her as

> a congenial type, and not irritable; calm; people say that she communicates a special serenity; a quiet type, shy. At home she isn't the type of person who screams and shouts. She likes to finish things, doesn't like to leave ends undone, and has to be organized. Pedantic, everything must be on time, things shouldn't be dragged out. If something is left undone—it disturbs her. She doesn't like to sit around idly. Since she became ill she was afraid of sicknesses. Her mother had died six years ago and her father was now dependent on Lily who had to do everything for him. It is like running two households. If a problem comes up, her father simply telephones her. She has

a brother with cerebral palsy who has been in an institution for the past four years. This preyed on her conscience, but her brother has adapted well. She has worked as a kindergarten teacher's aide for the past twenty-two years. The work is with small groups. She has close family ties—cousins her age—a social framework. They are more friends than family. The husband is helpful. He took care of her when she was sick, took her to doctors. He used to say that she didn't take care of herself, running around all the time. Childhood: Was very attached to her father. She was her grandmother's first granddaughter. Spoiled by grandmother, aunts, and uncles who were always around. At the peak of her sickness she didn't function at all. All she wanted to do was sleep. Every little thing was too much for her to accomplish. Her aunt used to come in and cook for her. Her daughter also helped. She didn't tell her father so as not to make him worry. Four years ago, in the course of a routine examination, she was diagnosed with a dermatological fungus. This hadn't bothered her and she was unaware of its existence. She was treated with a cream, which caused a localized itch followed by a serious infection of the entire area. It became a serious problem. The itch used to wake her up in the middle of sleep; it really used to make her jump up. She was treated with antibiotics continuously for eight months until she got sick and the treatment was stopped. Her diet included vegetables, fruit, milk products, and alcohol. Not particularly thirsty; suffers more from the cold. Seems calm, rational, very matter-of-fact. A person who doesn't "make a big fuss" out of things.

In contrast to the previous case, this one illustrates the nature of the homeopathic interview, which does indeed afford a different approach to the diagnosis and understanding of illness. The exact nature of the physiological complaint was less important than the patient's personal history and habits. The homeopath told the group that the patient had been back for another consultation because a wedding was coming up in the family, a son had gone away to college, and she had subsequently felt less than well during the past two weeks. She was concerned because she didn't know when it was going to end. She received homeopathic treatment, which did not help her, and so the dosage was changed. The patient stopped taking Prozac. She returned again after a couple of weeks complaining of a slight cough and weakness in the shoulders. She was treated with a placebo (not enough time had elapsed to allow for more homeopathic medicine), and is feeling fine.

The participants expressed some discomfort at the report of using a placebo. This was not verbally expressed, but evident in meaningful looks exchanged, gesticulation by Dr. Nadler, and a throat being cleared. The homeopath assumed a defiant, defensive look, pressing her lips together and raising her chin. This lack of ease can be understood in terms of conventional medicine's discomfort with the use of placebo, from an ethical as well as a therapeutic point of view. Curing with placebo somewhat defies the claim that homeopathic substances were active in themselves and their efficacy was not due to suggestion. The homeopath had perhaps inadvertently proved the opposite.

Conventional doctors have often, somewhat derogatorily, suggested that the placebo effect can provide an explanation for the success of NCM therapies. In response, NCM therapists have claimed that even if there were a placebo effect, there was nothing wrong with this as "placebo is the purest form of cure there is—it is the body healing itself." One MD present asked the practitioner whether she had weighed the patient at the outset of treatment and at its end. This, he said, would have constituted quantifiable proof of cure. This indicates that the medically trained mind is on the lookout for something that can be measured and communicated to conventional medicine; the therapist's (or patient's) subjective report of improvement was not sufficient.

In general, jokingly, the patient was described as a "good" patient at the clinic. Her repeated visits were not only an indication of compliance, which would lead to recovery, but also a source of income for the clinic. Antibiotics were discussed as the source of the patient's problems and Dr. Binnaker suggested that the clinic establish an on-call advisory body that patients could contact if the necessity to take antibiotics should arise. In this case a qualified MD could assess the situation, provide a second opinion, and discuss the matter with the patient's family practitioner in an attempt to prevent unnecessary use of antibiotics. This idea was somewhat political in essence, as it afforded the MDs an additional advantage over the non-MD practitioners and also opened a channel of professional discourse between the clinic and conventional MDs that the patients were supposed to initiate. Although everyone agreed that this was a good idea, nothing operative materialized.

Discussion on the second case was sparse because it did not represent a common problem, which everybody could identify with and participate in, such as the patient who "won't" get well. The fact that all others present at the meeting were not homeopaths precluded discussion on the particular choice of medication (one of 2,000 options), dosage, or the use of placebo. Once again, as in the previous case, conventional medicine constituted the common frame of reference and the only response offered from the forum was the manner in which other modalities could treat the problem.

Whereas the case study presented by the MD constituted a conventional write-up with an NCM solution, the homeopathic write-up presented by the non-MD practitioner provided a somewhat different description of the illness process. This manner of describing, seeing, and ascribing probably does constitute an alternative "hearing" of illness and cure. However, in the context of the staff meeting, the *dominant* gaze was still that of conventional medicine. This probably resulted from the fact that a number of different therapists practicing a variety of alternative therapies were present at the meeting. The very different philosophical bases, cultural origins, and history of these therapies made the discussion difficult. It is, however, interesting to observe that a general discourse of holism, individualism, and subjectivity did not replace the conventional medical view as a unifying factor. The most natural, common point of reference was that of conventional, scientific medicine. Diagnosis was always presented in terms of conventional medicine, along with the particular treatment available in the different disciplines.

Magic

In addition to the use of scientific medicine as a frame of reference, another—seemingly opposite—theme was present in the discussions—namely, magic. Practitioners and doctors alike took endless pains to stress that cure was a result of cooperation, hard work, and a long haul. There was no hocus-pocus involved. However, magic and the supernatural, introduced by means of humor, seemed to provide an ever-present subtext. For example, one day at the clinic a nurse pointed out to an MD homeopath a beautiful bunch of garden-fresh roses on the receptionist's table. "Put in a few drops of homeopathic essence and they will live forever," he jokingly remarked. At staff meetings a tradition developed of presenting the birthday people of the month with a "rescue remedy." This remedy, in the form of an aromatic essence in a small, brown medicinal bottle was supposed to provide instant aid in case of mental or physical crisis.

Although I have already mentioned the practitioners' awareness that promising too much would have negative repercussions and culminate in disappointment and noncompliance, such claims of potency were hard to resist. This was generally evident in interviews published in the media, and was also observed at another staff meeting in which a prominent clinical dietician took responsibility for the case exposition. Instead of discussing an actual case, the dietician presented an article from a scientific journal that discussed the use of food as an emergency, short-term method of clinical intervention.

The dietician claimed that although dietary changes were being employed as a means of healing or prevention, it was a mistake to see these changes solely as a long-term method. In her opinion, food could serve as emergency medicine. She claimed that as a result of emergency nutrition a bout of flu lasted for "half a day." She also recounted the story of a friend's hospitalization due to a heart attack. Although her friend was placed in intensive care, she claimed that giving her antioxidant vegetable juices at the height of the crisis minimized the subsequent damage to her blood vessels. This claim brings to mind the "magic bullet" approach characteristic of the claims and expectations of conventional medicine. The magic of the alternative, therefore, lies not only in its gentle, natural, gradual essence, but also in its ability to harness the power of nature to achieve immediate, dramatic cure. While such reference to "magic" existed, it did not occupy the same status as the reference to biomedicine.

Chapter 4

The Patients: Group Profile and Patterns of Use

NCM's popularity has been on the rise for the last decade. For example, Eisenberg's (1993) study of a national sample in the United States showed that 34% of the respondents had used at least one NCM therapy in the past year. A replication of this study in 1998 found that the number had risen to 42.1%. In Europe, a similar increase in NCM consumption is apparent. Menges (1994) reports that between 1981 and 1990, the number of NCM users in the Netherlands had risen by 0.3% per annum, while the number of people visiting an MD who provided alternative treatment rose in the same period by 1%. According to Fisher (1994), the number of people who had visited an NCM practitioner in the past twelve months in the United Kingdom rose from one in seven in 1985 to almost one in four in 1991. The use of homeopathy in France (the most popular NCM method there) rose from 16% of the population in 1982 to 29% in 1987, and 36% in 1992.

A study conducted in Israel by Bernstein and Shuval (1997) showed that use of NCM therapies is quite widespread; 6% of the population over the age of forty-five reported consultation with an NCM practitioner in the course of the previous year. An additional survey conducted by the Brandman Institute (1993) showed that 20% of the respondents stated that either they or an immediate family member had consulted an NCM practitioner in the past year.

In general, surveys that have indicated widespread use of NCM modalities have focused on the demographic profile of NCM users, the medical problems commonly treated by NCM, and reasons for its use (e.g., dissatisfaction with CM, the doctor–patient relationship, or fear of CM side effects). However, the attitudes held by consumers of NCM therapies have not been the target of much empirical research, and information has been largely of a conjectural or qualitative nature. In the Introduction, I proposed four theoretical categories that offered explanations for public recourse to NCM. The first two approaches, "modernization" and "limited dissatisfaction," explained the recourse to NCM as a reflection of traditional values or as a second resort to conventional biomedicine, respectively. These approaches could not, however, explain the increasing popularity of NCM as a therapeutic option. A third approach, called "general dissatisfaction," focused on the use of NCM as an expression of counterculture while the fourth approach seemed to indicate that NCM had become part of the therapeutic options open to a public that was now choosing among conventional and nonconventional modalities in a consumerist-oriented fashion, maximizing what was perceived as the particular benefit of each modality.

Cultural Outlook and the Use of NCM

Sparse empirical data exist on the part played by a specific cultural outlook in the decision to use NCM, and much is of a theoretical, perhaps even conjectural nature. Ursula Sharma (1992: 204), for example, argued that "the explicit pursuit of cultural ideas about health care did not enter into their (the patients') stories of the decision that led them into the consulting room of the complementary therapist in the first place." However, in health-seeking behavior, it has been pointed out that the patient's social mileu, perceived as a "therapeutic community" (Kleinman, 1980), is instrumental in the decision to seek help as well as evaluate the outcome of treatment. The impetus to seek alternative treatment, or view it as a viable option, starts well before the actual consultation with the practitioner. Recourse to NCM can thus be a reflection of a more general lifestyle. It has been suggested (Bakx, 1991; Cant and Calnan, 1991; Douglas, 1994) that the growing interest in NCM is part of a general, postmodern outlook that not only rejects science and technology, but subscribes to a "green," New Age, and "back-to-nature" ideology. Other aspects characteristic of this outlook are preoccupation with the body, fascination with the "cultural other," and an attraction to the esoteric or supernatural.

Mary Douglas (1994: 25), for example, states that therapeutic choice is indeed cultural in essence: "Alternative medicine, is, in short, a cultural alternative to western, philosophical traditions." Douglas thus assumes the existence of a coherent "cultural type":

> We would expect people who show a strong preference for holistic medicine to be negative to the kind of culture in which the other kind of medicine belongs. If they have made the choice for a gentler, more spiritual medicine, they will be making the same choice in other contexts, dietary, ecological, as well as medical. Their choice of alternative medicine will not be an isolated preference, uncoordinated with other values upheld by the patient (ibid., p. 32).

Quantitative studies that focused on cultural aspects of NCM use were inconclusive. For example, Astin (1998) explored whether a group characterized as "cultural creatives" was more likely to use NCM. These individuals were prone to a holistic orientation to health, a commitment to environmentalism and feminism, an interest in spirituality and personal growth philosophy, self-actualization and self-expression, as well as a love of the foreign and exotic. However, the fact that all these attributes were measured as a basket of values and not individually did not afford much insight into the so-called cultural type that consumed NCM. Furnham and Forrey (1994) explored the connection between specific cultural characteristics and the propensity to use NCM. The items examined were: an ecologically aware lifestyle, an interest in the body, the environment, food, and use of natural products. Their data showed that NCM users were more likely to be vegetarians and shop in health food stores. The other items were not supported.

In order to achieve deeper understanding about the part played by cultural beliefs in the decision to use NCM, I decided to interview patients who had visited the NCM clinic described in the previous chapter. A definite trend did not emerge from these interviews. Some patients were indeed eager to have their problem rephrased and treated in nonconventional terms, as illustrated by the following two stories selected from the interviews.

A young woman, a graduate student in psychology, had been suffering from back pain, which radiated down her leg. At the orthopedic clinic, to which she had been referred, no anatomical reason had been found for her complaint and she had been told that she probably had a rheumatic disease. In an interview with me she was adamant that "a 'rheumatic disease' is no diagnosis! I want to know what's wrong with me—what is causing all this. On one hand I feel silly at the orthopedic clinic among all those people who limp and look really sick, but on the other hand, no one has helped me. And all the time I couldn't help thinking: If only there were a Chinese doctor or something like that around here, I'm sure he'd be able to find an explanation for what is happening with me. Why it's happening." In this case the patient was very eager to have her problem explained by another paradigm. Conventional medicine had not offered a satisfactory explanation for her pain, beyond the fact that anatomical malfunction was not detected. She viewed alternative medicine as being able to provide both explanation and cure for her problem, and was only too willing to adopt it. She was indeed very willing to entertain an alternative explanation for her problem, one not necessarily expressed in biomedical terms and etiology. In her view Chinese medicine would be able to provide this etiology.

Another patient voiced a similar opinion: "I like to think differently, I admire original thought, and I thought that was what you people did at the clinic—try and get at the root of the problem. To look for an explanation as to why it has happened, and not just try and treat the symptoms superficially or compensate chemically for what the body lacks. I thought you had unconventional thoughts on new directions in healing." This patient was disappointed by the somewhat conventional manner in which his thyroid problem had been dealt with in the complementary clinic. He was told to continue with conventional medication and offered "extra support" by means of herbal remedies with a view to perhaps gradually decreasing the dosage of the conventional drug. The quest by patients for a different language or etiology of sickness expresses something that—as we saw in the previous chapter—was absent from the staff discussions at the clinic. These meetings, as I have illustrated, supported a predominantly conventional view of illness and healing.

These two stories are typical of differentiation, counterculture [in Douglas's (1994) terminology] and possibly "cultural creativeness," as Astin (1998) calls it. However, this was not the whole picture. Many other patients were not happy at all with New Age alternatives at the clinic. In fact, they found them offensive. One such respondent, who received treatment lying on the floor on a mat instead of a regular couch, complained to me that "the treatment was enough to make you sick. It made me feel worse, my neck ached and ached." Another patient, commenting on classical homeopathy, said: "The granules were a lot of nonsense. How can one dose cure anything?" Yet another patient, who had received reflexology treatment, complained that the therapist lit a candle before treatment and said this would help the healing process. The patient said: "I don't want 'healing' and I don't want reflexology—the therapist didn't even look at my hands—how can all this make me better?" It therefore appears that the cultural outlook of NCM patients is not uniform. Some patients are in pursuit of a cultural New Age experience, while others are not (Fadlon, 2004a). In the attempt to move beyond this variation and detect a definite trend, I decided to administer a questionnaire to a large sample of patients.

For this purpose, the concerns, attitudes, and preferences of 304 patients attending the NCM clinic were examined with regard to the theoretical issues and ethnographic material described in the previous chapters. In order to discover whether NCM patients could indeed be characterized by a unique outlook, an additional 322 questionnaires were distributed to patients attending two conventional outpatient clinics: an orthopedic outpatient clinic at the same hospital as the NCM clinic (155 respondents) and an allergy clinic at another hospital (167 respondents). Questionnaires were administered to all these groups between 1995 and 1996 with the intent of comparing the attitudes of the NCM clinic patients with those of the CM (conventional medicine) clinic patients.

Preliminary statistical analysis of the two groups revealed that many of the CM clinic patients had had some experience with NCM methods. Indeed, 20% of the patients attending a conventional outpatient clinic said that at present they were being treated by NCM, and an additional 13% said that in the past they had received NCM treatments. The use of NCM methods therefore appears to be quite widespread—33% of the patients at the conventional clinics had some kind of experience with NCM. Due to these results, which showed that many CM clinic patients were also NCM users, I decided to reshuffle the groups and create two new groups for comparison: those who had **never** used NCM as opposed to those who had **ever** used NCM, irrespective of the clinic where they had been recruited to answer the questionnaire.

But before we proceed to this new frame of comparison, I would like to describe the common patterns of recourse to medical treatment identified at all three clinics. As we have seen, 20% of the patients visiting a conventional clinic were receiving NCM treatment concomitantly. A similar pattern of dual use characterized the patients attending the NCM clinic. Among them, 41% were still using conventional methods and remedies for their condition. It is interesting to note the *dual system strategy* adopted by patients at both the NCM and regular clinics. This finding is important as it seems to indicate that many patients do not feel that they have to choose between the two systems, but rather combine them according to necessity or choice. In other words, these findings seem to refute differentiation and validate domestication. Dual use has also been reported by Bernstein and Shuval (1997), who found that 39% of their sample were seeing conventional doctors and NCM practitioners at the same time. We now move our frame of reference from the comparison between the NCM and CM clinics to a comparison between those patients who had had some kind of experience with NCM to those who had never used it.

Sociodemographic Characteristics and Health Problems

In terms of sociodemographic characteristics (see Table 1), the two groups under comparison (214 patients who had never used NCM as opposed to 412 who had had some kind of treatment with NCM) seem to differ in two main aspects. There were more women (60.4% vs. 44.4%) among the NCM users in comparison with those who had never received NCM treatment, and the former group was also considerably older than the latter (43.7 vs. 33.3 years, on average). Other differences between the groups, such as marital status and number of children, may be attributed to the age difference. No significant differences between the groups were found in terms of ethnic origin, occupation, education, or extent of religiosity. The medical problems of the patients using NCM (see Table 2) indicate that NCM users are suffering from a more chronic type of problem such as pain, allergies, and stress-related complaints.

Patients' Attitudes toward Biomedicine

When do patients think it is appropriate to turn to NCM? Table 3 provides a statistical answer to this question. Not surprisingly, more patients who had ever used NCM (32%) thought it was appropriate to resort to NCM even before trying conventional treatment for a certain problem. In fact, this was the most frequent answer chosen in reply to the question. In contrast, fewer respondents among those who never used NCM (10%) expressed this attitude toward the issue. The most frequent answer chosen by those who never used NCM (32%) was "it

Table 1. Sociodemographic Characteristics

Sociodemographic characteristic	Never used NCM $N = 214$	NCM users $N = 412$	Difference statistic
Gender (percent women)	44.4	60.4	$\chi^2 = 14.7$***
Age (mean)	33.2	43.7	$t = 7.9$***
Ethnic origin (percent Sephardi)	11.2	13.1	$\chi^2 = .5$
Education level (%)			
Primary school	6.2	5.9	$\chi^2 = .5$
Vocational high school	18.2	20.8	
Matriculation high school	42.1	36	
College	13.9	13.7	
University (BA)	17.2	18.4	
University (MA)	2.4	3.9	
University (PhD)	0	1.2	
% Married	46.3	66.8	$\chi^2 = 24.6$***
Number of children (mean)	1.3	2.1	$t = 5.45$***
Religiosity (%)			
Secular	58	62.8	$\chi^2 = .5$
Traditional	30.2	27.1	
Orthodox	11.8	10.1	

***$p<0.001$

Table 2. Health Problems

Health problem	Never used NCM $N - 214$	NCM users $N - 412$	Difference statistic
Complaint type (%)			
Psychosomatic and stress problems	2.8	20.4	$\chi^2 = 35.4$***
Orthopedic pains	36.9	39.2	$\chi^2 = .3$
Allergies, respiration and skin	46.7	28.4	$\chi^2 = 20.9$***
Other	12.2	20.6	$\chi^2 = 4.4$**
Duration of condition (mean)	3.7	3.8	$t = 1.3$

**$p<0.01$
***$p<0.001$

depends on the condition." This was also the second most frequent answer chosen by the other group (29%). All in all, the findings of Table 3 support the hypothesis that those who never used NCM are more conformist with the hegemony of biomedicine, while those who had ever used NCM appear to be more subversive. However, the fact that the most frequent answer given by those who never used NCM was "it depends on the condition" (32%) shows that their "conformity" is pragmatic and depends on the success/failure of biomedical treatment. The fact that 29% of NCM users said that "it depends on the condition" and 22% said "only after conventional methods" may also reflect a situation of limited dissatisfaction with biomedicine. The fact that more NCM users supported using NCM before CM could also be a result of successful experience with a certain NCM modality resulting in the realization that for certain problems NCM might indeed be the better choice. The hypothesis of NCM as an ideological counterculture (i.e., general dissatisfaction) would have arguably been supported if a vast majority of NCM users had chosen the first answer, thus affording NCM full-fledged priority. What the table shows is that there is no clear-cut priority in either group and that the situation is quite negotiable.

As expected, NCM users were less satisfied with conventional treatment of their condition ($M = 2.4$) than those who never used NCM ($M = 2.8$). It is, however, interesting to note that both groups of patients were satisfied with the general treatment received from the conventional doctor. This dissatisfaction with the outcome of conventional medical treatment does not necessarily extend to include its representative—the conventional MD, who was generally afforded a high rating in terms of communication and quality of treatment, as

Table 3. Attitudes toward the Hegemony of Biomedicine (numbers represent % of positive replies)

It's right to turn to alternative methods:	Never used NCM	NCM users
1. Even before conventional methods	10	32
2. Only after conventional methods	29	22
3. It depends on the condition	32	29
4. Don't know	29	17
Total	100	100

$\chi^2(3_{n=606}) = 42.7, p < .001$

Table 4 shows. In any event, there were no significant differences in the level of satisfaction with the MD. Most important, patients from both groups thought it was very important that nonconventional treatment be provided by an MD. Agreement with this stance was actually slightly stronger among NCM users (an average of 3.7 compared to 3.5 among those who never used NCM). This interesting and unpredicted finding suggests that NCM users—the very group that could have been characterized as subversive and countercultural—actually conforms to the hegemony of biomedicine by preferring the nonconventional treatment to be overseen by a doctor. Taken together with the limited dissatisfaction with CM implied in the findings of Table 3, and the general satisfaction with the conventional therapist, the overall attitude of NCM users appears to distinguish pragmatically between the nature of the therapy and its benefit. The findings support the view that NCM users do not generally protest against biomedicine, but rather against a particular unsuccessful biomedical treatment.

Table 4. Satisfaction with Conventional Treatment and Practitioner

	Never used NCM	NCM users	Difference statistic
Are you generally satisfied with your health condition? (1—very dissatisfied, 4—very satisfied)	2.8	2.5	$t = 4.1$***
Satisfaction w/ conv. treatment (1—very dissatisfied, 4—very satisfied)	2.8	2.4	$t = 6.7$***
Satisfaction w/ doctor (1—very dissatisfied, 5—very satisfied)	4.2	4.1	$t = 1.1$
Satisfaction w/ doctor in terms of communication	4.1	4	$t = .5$
Satisfaction w/ quality of treatment	4.0	3.8	$t = 2.2$*
It is important that an MD provides the nonconventional treatment (1—not important at all, 4—very important)	3.5	3.7	$t = 2.8$**

*$p<0.05$
**$p<0.01$
***$p<0.001$

Cultural Outlook and Practices

The findings in Table 5 do not support the contention that using NCM is part of a general predisposition to New Age trends. No significant differences were apparent between the two groups except on the one item related to receiving treatment from a religious healer. Significantly more NCM users said that they had approached a religious healer for treatment and this finding could perhaps be explained within the context of activism (willingness to "try everything") characteristic of NCM users. About 40% of both groups said they believed in miracles, a finding that supports the view that religious healing does not play a predominant role nor does it constitute part of an alternative ideology. Overall, no distinct linkage could be established with regard to CM patients being more 'rational' and NCM patients being more involved in New Age philosophies. This possible linkage was further examined through various statements comparing the ideological worldviews that appear in Table 6.

Replies to the ideological statements appearing in Table 6 indicate that NCM users are somewhat more wary of science than their CM counterparts. Significantly more NCM patients believed that reliance on science implied ignoring emotion and intuition. They were also more skeptical that science would ultimately find a solution to problems. These more critical attitudes toward science, however, did not automatically lead to an alternative worldview. There was no difference between the groups in their evaluation of Far Eastern culture. Indeed, both groups thought that there was something to be learned from both America and the Far East. This most definitely goes against the common belief that NCM users have a particular affinity with the Far East and its cultural traditions.

Table 5. Esoteric Beliefs (numbers represent % of 'yes')

	Never used NCM	NCM users	Difference statistic
Do you believe in astrology?	28	24.9	$\chi^2 = .7$
Did you ever approach a religious healer for treatment?	15.2	25.7	$\chi^2 = 8.9**$
Do you believe in miracles?	40.4	39.5	$\chi^2 = .1$
Did you ever use crystals or "lucky stones"?	14.6	20.3	$\chi^2 = 3$

**$p<0.01$

Table 6. Statements Concerning Ideological Worldviews

	Never used NCM	NCM users	Difference statistic
Do you agree with the following statements? (1—disagree completely, 4—agree completely)			
"We rely too much on science and technology while ignoring emotion and intuition"	3.2	3.4	$t = 2.9$**
"Science generally causes more damage than benefit"	2.2	2.4	$t = 1.7$
"Science will eventually find a solution for all our problems"	2.9	2.7	$t = 2.8$**
"I often yearn to leave the city for a healthier lifestyle"	3.6	3.6	$t = .4$
"We have a lot to learn from traditional Far East culture"	3.3	3.4	$t = 1.3$
"We have a lot to learn from American culture"	3.1	3.4	$t = 3$**

**$p<0.01$

Table 7. Consumerist Practices

	Never used NCM	NCM users	Difference statistic
Do you agree with the following statements (1—never, 4—always)			
"It is important to buy only ozone-friendly products"	3.2	3.3	$t = .8$
"When buying food products, I check for conserving chemicals"	2.8	2.9	$t = 1.6$
"I am willing to pay more for organic food"	2.8	3.0	$t = 1.7$
"I often visit organic food stores"	1.9	2.4	$t = 4.4$***
Readiness for lifestyle change that would promote relief of symptoms (1—none, 5—very much)	3.6	3.8	$t = 2.3$*
Are you interested in media reports on health subjects? (1—not at all, 5—very much)	3.6	3.8	$t = 2.6$**

*$p<0.05$
**$p<0.01$
***$p<0.001$

Table 8. Views of the Body (unless noted otherwise, numbers represent averages on a scale of 1 [don't agree] to 4 [agree completely])

	Never used NCM	NCM users	Difference statistic
I am usually aware of changes in my physical condition	3.3	3.3	$t = .9$
It is important that a person maintains a young look	3.3	3.3	$t = .8$
Have you ever had cosmetic surgery? (% of 'yes')	3.3	4.2	$\chi^2 = .3$
Were you ever on a diet in order to lose weight (1—never, 5—I'm on a diet right now)	2.1	2.3	$t = 2.3*$
Do you think that your physical condition is influenced by your mental state?	3.0	3.1	$t = 2.1*$
Do you take vitamins (1—no, 5—every day)	1.8	2	$t = 1.8$

*$p<0.05$

A prevalent ideological image linked to NCM patients is their supposed interest in the body, fitness, and a healthier lifestyle. This possible linkage was examined in Tables 7 and 8. Whereas Table 7 shows that both CM and NCM users are discerning consumers, significantly more NCM patients prefer organic food stores and are interested in media reports on health subjects. They are also more willing than their CM counterparts to make an effort and change their lifestyle if this were to promote their health and well-being. However, similar attitudes are also characteristic of CM patients. Table 8 further illustrates that there is no real difference between the two groups. Very slight differences exist in the frequency of dieting and the awareness of a mind-body connectedness. The questionnaires therefore did not provide any clear support for differentiation.

Similar findings are discussed by McGregor and Peay (1996), who found that Australian patients who use NCM do not hold a less positive view of conventional medicine. They characterize these patients as:

> Less prepared to accept the outcomes that conventional treatment was able to provide... coupled with their higher assessment of their own control over their health... [they are] a

group characterized by a greater determination to make their own decisions about the best ways in which to deal with their own health problems (1996: 1326).

NCM users in Israel therefore emerge from the questionnaires as pragmatic consumers. A similar conclusion is discussed by Kelner and Wellman (1997: 211), who characterized NCM users as "individuals who have essentially taken their health and well-being into their own hands ... acting as concerned consumers rather than compliant patients." The pragmatism of NCM users is manifested in "smart consumerism," that is, "choosing specific kinds of practitioners for particular problems ... chiropractors for backaches, naturopaths for colds, Reiki practitioners for emotional stress, acupuncture for allergies ... many use multiple therapies concurrently" (Kelner and Wellman, 1997: 211). The empirical data on the Israeli cohort show that although some differences between the two groups do indeed exist, these differences seem to point toward behavior that can be defined as active consumerism, rather than deep cultural, ideological differences. These findings support my claim that domestication can be seen as the driving force behind the popularization of NCM in a number of contexts.

The Convergence of Statistics and Ethnography

The statistical data indicate that NCM users cannot be characterized by a specific sociodemographic profile. They do not belong to a specific ethnic group and are not differentiated by either occupation or education. The "modernization approach" therefore cannot explain recourse to NCM. Its users are not less educated, they do not fill a less prestigious occupational role, and they do not belong to a specific ethnic group.

The "second resort" approach suggested that patients were likely to turn to NCM following disappointment with conventional medicine. This suggestion is partly supported by my findings. Patients attending the NCM clinic were significantly less satisfied with conventional medical treatment than their counterparts. However, the finding that 32% of those at the NCM clinic and 10% of those at the CM clinic felt that it was appropriate to turn to NCM *even before* all options in the field of CM had been exhausted indicates that this approach cannot entirely explain the recourse to NCM.

The third approach ("general dissatisfaction") suggested that NCM users could be characterized by a consistent New Age cultural profile.

This approach was also refuted by the statistical findings. Patients at the NCM clinic, although dissatisfied with conventional treatment, preferred that an MD provide NCM treatment. From the point of view of cultural outlook, NCM users could indeed be characterized by slightly more skepticism toward science and professed awareness of a body-mind connection. They did not, however, differ from their CM counterparts in their interest in mystical and New Age activities. The emerging picture therefore refutes the construction of a specific, consistent cultural profile of the NCM consumer, as suggested by Douglas (1994).

A significant and consistent finding was that NCM patients evaluated their physical and mental condition as less positive than those attending the CM clinic (see Table 2). Because of this more negative, subjective evaluation, NCM patients were probably more willing to invest time and effort in treating their health and changing their lifestyle to achieve better health. Forty-one percent of the NCM patients, however, also reported that they were still using conventional methods to deal with their ailment. This dual pattern of use was also reported by Bernstein and Shuval (1997) and Sirois and Gick (2002). Kelner and Wellman (1997) similarly reported that patients tend to choose from an array of therapies, moving between conventional and nonconventional modalities according to the specific ailment. These findings indicate that processes of domestication have successfully rendered NCM methods a non-exotic, "matter-of-fact" choice in the field of health consumption. The fact that consumers use both methods concomitantly or move between the methods indicates that recourse to NCM now exists as a viable choice, as suggested in the fourth approach, that of medical pluralism and active consumerism.

Not surprisingly, NCM users were less satisfied with the outcome of conventional treatment. Dissatisfaction was, however, limited (to the particular medical treatment used) rather than general (toward biomedicine as a whole). While preferring that a medical doctor remains in supervision, NCM users also expressed a greater tendency to experiment with nonconventional methods. I explained this tendency as reflecting active consumerism rather than alternative ideology. The limited dissatisfaction of NCM users probably makes them more amenable to trying out new therapies, depending on their condition. The fact that more NCM users suffer chronic pain probably promotes their motivation to seek new therapies when conventional biomedicine has failed to offer a remedy. Their search for a cure is tentative and pragmatic. It is not a quest for an alternative, but rather an attempt to find personal alleviation of symptoms. According to the statistical findings, NCM users are more likely to visit health food stores or more prone to dieting. This interest in health is not the outcome of neurotic, hypersensitive, or "complaining" behavior that might be labeled (by biomedicine) as psychologically morbid. On the contrary, it appears to be the behavior of active and empowered consumers. The consumerist behavior and attitudes of NCM users, illustrated this time by means of quantitative methods, can be perceived as both promoting the assimilation of NCM and a result of its domestication.

Chapter 5

Dissemination:
The Popular Discourse of NCM

It was a well-established fact at the complementary clinic that I studied that following media coverage the secretaries were inundated with telephone calls from the public. The benefits of the media were well appreciated at the clinic.[1] For example, during one of the staff meetings the decrease in the number of patients consulting the clinic was noted. One of the therapists (non-MD) asked: "Well, can't we get any press coverage?" The MD in charge of the clinic responded that he had been "buttering up" a number of journalists for quite some time, and that results could be expected soon.

The staff at the clinic was also well aware that the media could be used in the inter- and intraprofessional struggle for recognition and legitimacy. By gaining popular support for NCM, and increasing public knowledge and demand, practitioners were, in fact, conducting a professional campaign for assimilation. Often unable to find common grounds for discourse with the medical profession or medico-legal establishment, practitioners of NCM were actually directly communicating with the public through the popular press, thereby creating a demand for their services. This was an attempt to control the process by which NCM was perceived by the public.

Whereas NCM thrives on publicity, the medical establishment has regarded the role of the media with mixed feelings. The Israeli Medical Association has recommended that the same restrictions forbidding doctors to advertise themselves to the public should also be enforced for NCM practitioners, whether they are MDs or not. This stance recognizes the challenge posed by free competition between NCM and biomedicine and the power inherent in direct communication with the public concerning the advantages of certain treatments.

Interprofessional Discourse in the Public Arena

The exchange of professional knowledge generally occurs in professional publications and interprofessional discussions. The results of these scientific discussions are then usually simplified for the public and appear in more general, popular publications. In this manner the medical or scientific community has control over the knowledge that reaches the public as it is first evaluated and discussed among peers (Hilgartner, 1990). In the case of the media, NCM practitioners assume the role of experts in their field and directly disseminate information to the public that has not been evaluated or approved by conventional medicine or accepted scientific procedure. This is particularly interesting when the disseminators are qualified MDs who practice NCM, which renders the message all the more powerful. In this manner the hegemony but not the authority of biomedicine are undermined as these practitioners use their authority as biomedical physicians to promote NCM. These NCM practitioners, who are also qualified MDs, act as "cultural entrepreneurs" or "cultural brokers" (Hannerz, 1996) who "carve out their own niche, find their own market segment, by developing a product more specifically attuned to the characteristics of their local consumers. . . . These local entrepreneurs have the advantage of knowing their territory. Their particular asset is cultural competence, cultural sensibility. Through their roots in local forms of life, they sense which concerns and tastes can be translated into market shares" (p. 74). The media thus becomes a postmodern arena in which knowledge claims and therapeutic claims are evaluated and disseminated.

Kleinman (1980) has already commented that "it is the lay, non-professional, non-specialist, popular culture arena in which illness is first defined and health care activities initiated" (1980: 50). The case of NCM in the media fully supports Kleinmen's view that

> After patients receive treatment, they return to the popular sector to evaluate it and decide what to do next. The popular sector is the nexus of the boundaries between the various sectors; it contains the points of entrance into, exit from, and

interaction between the different sectors. The popular sector interacts with each of the other sectors, whereas they are frequently isolated from each other. The customary view is that professionals organize health care for lay people. But typically lay people activate their health care by deciding when and whom to consult, whether or not to comply, when to switch between treatment alternatives, whether care is effective, and whether they are satisfied with its quality. In this sense, the popular sector functions as the chief source and most immediate determinant of care (p. 51).

The media acts as a type of virtual therapeutic community in which NCM practitioners provide a new vocabulary for defining health and illness. They also directly communicate with the public, leaning on medical authority (in the case of MD NCM practitioners) and promote knowledge and therapeutic claims that may not be scientifically acceptable according to the criteria of evidence-based medicine. This is probably the reason why the medical association is so anxious to extend the media restraints that apply to the medical community to NCM practitioners as well. Giddens (1994) has indeed commented that "information produced by specialists (including scientific knowledge) can no longer be wholly confined to specific groups, but becomes routinely interpreted and acted upon by lay individuals in the course of their everyday actions" (1994:7). These "lay interpretations" are directed by expositions of NCM in the press as we will see in this chapter.

Should we expect the hierarchical division between biomedicine and NCM to diminish and collapse in a way similar to the distinction between high culture and mass culture as a result of the media's involvement? This would probably be the prediction of sociologists who have equated "the postmodern" with processes of dedifferentiation and deregulation (Turner, 1992). Such a prediction, however, has not yet materialized, although studies conducted on the representation of medicine in the media are as yet inconclusive. Karpf (1988 in Bury and Gabe, 1994), for example, presents a historic view of the relationship between the media and medicine and shows how the medical establishment retained its dominance in the 1930s and 1940s by withholding information from the public. Although subsequent years were characterized by a more open relationship with the media and challenges to the medical establishment were posed by feminist and consumerist movements, Karpf concludes that biomedical dominance will remain intact. Bury and Gabe (1994) challenge this conclusion and claim that the media act as carriers and amplifiers of a more challenging position. Although the medical profession and the biomedical model of health and illness still hold considerable prestige in society, this position is under pressure. Williams and Calnan (1996) also conclude that the media serve a demystifying function, thereby challenging the hegemony of biomedicine. In the case of the representation of NCM in the media, it could be argued that while a process of demystification is instigated by practitioners of NCM in order to weaken the dominant position of CM, a parallel mystifying process is created around the therapeutic claims of NCM.

Lupton (1995) observed that an overlap between health values and aesthetic attributes is pertinent to the portrayal of NCM in the media. NCM is promoted through the media as an ideal situation of holistic self-realization in which body and soul are in harmony with each other as well as with the environment. Insecurities and feelings of disharmony, played out through the body, are evoked, only to be solved by NCM. This was also apparent in the Israeli media. For example, the issue of achieving a physical and mental state of harmony and balance often links NCM treatments such as Ayur Vedah massage or aromatherapy to health spas (*Yediot* 18.10.2000; *Yediot* 15.6.2000) In this manner health, aesthetics and NCM become part of the postmodern concern with the body enacted this time not in the gymnasium but in the spa.

The media provides a legitimate way for NCM to "bypass" the formalities of the biomedical establishment and address the public directly. NCM practitioners use this invaluable privilege quite successfully. The media was crucial in garnering public demand that in turn led to the incorporation of NCM within the confines of established medical institutions such as hospitals and health funds. The press also provides an arena in which representatives of conventional and nonconventional medicine can air their differences, vie for public attention, and conduct their interprofessional battles. The role of the media thus fulfills a significant role in the understanding of the domestication of NCM. In what follows I present findings based on textual analysis of 132 articles published in the daily Israeli press between 1991 and 2001. In general, the representation of medicine in the media can be divided into various formats such as government-sponsored advertising, commercial advertising, interviews and talk shows in which members of the public, the medical profession, or NCM practitioners air their views or grievances on a particular subject; documentary films, journalistic exposes, popular dramatic serials, and full-length features. The messages disseminated through these different platforms are often contradictory (Novelli, 1990). My focus on newspaper articles stems from the fact that these are the most accessible media platform available in Israel and present the opportunity to systematically explore the interaction between NCM and CM practitioners in the public arena. Moreover, the written press, in particular, served to cultivate a "community" or a social world in which patients could symbolically and vicariously, through identification with first-person accounts, evaluate their own health status and treatments already received.

The Narrative Formula of Dissemination

What follows is a narrative analysis of three stories in which a particular hybrid form of NCM that is at once familiar and exotic emerges. I argue that the creation of this hybrid renders NCM both attractive and acceptable to the public, and introduces a dialogue with conventional medicine. In the framework of this dialogue the hegemony, but not the authority, of biomedicine is challenged.

The three stories from which examples will be drawn highlight the underlying narrative formula of these media accounts (Berger, 1997). All narratives can be identified by several essential elements (Gergen and Gergen, 1988; Maines, 1993; Mitchel, 1981). The first element is that events must be selected from the past for purposes of focus and commentary. This is achieved in the articles through the presentation of an "illness story." Second, these events must be transformed into story elements. This is contrived through the use of plot, setting, and characterization that confer structure, meaning, and context on the events selected. In the interviews, the illness story comprises a plot that moves (in retrospective) through three classical stages—exposition (of the patient's situation), entanglement (a health problem that could not be treated conventionally), and denouement (the cure offered by NCM and, most important, its ultimate integration into biomedicine).

A common feature of the three stories to be examined is their multifaceted exposition as a narrative within a narrative. The story of the physician is as interesting as the story of the patient. Both have "overcome adversity" and "weakness of body and spirit" in the form of a symbolic journey that culminates in enlightenment, cure, and tranquility. Beyond the oppositions observable in these texts, it is equally interesting to note the fusion of opposites inherent in them. This fusion of opposites constitutes what could perhaps epitomize the essence of domestication.

Magic Moments

Story 1: If I Get Pricked, It Won't Hurt

This story, which appeared under the title "If I get pricked, it won't hurt" (*Maariv* 5.15.1996), was accompanied by a photograph of one of the two doctors interviewed. Dr. P., with a Chinese-style moustache, was shown holding a figurine marked with meridians. The article opened with a dramatic narrative.

> In the last two months of first grade, Lee spent more time at home than at school. "The child, all of six and a half years, consumed more antibiotics than candy," says her mother. "We went from one doctor to another with repeated throat and ear infections, accompanied by high fever. When we had given up on the sick fund's ability to help, we turned to private E.N.T. doctors. She had her eardrum pierced but to no avail. The doctors talked about a tonsillectomy and implantation of grommets in her ears. The child started losing weight. I started to panic.
>
> A friend told me that there was an alternative medicine clinic at the General Hospital. My husband said that medicinal herbs and all that kind of mumbo jumbo belonged to primitive tribes. But when the doctors prescribed antibiotics once again and I saw how weak the child had become, a shadow of her former self, I insisted we consult the alternative medicine clinic. I decided that if an alternative existed in the framework of a hospital, it was worth a try and so I rang up the clinic and look at her now. Blossoming."

This narrative contains the seemingly irreconcilable opposites of mumbo jumbo and medical science, skepticism (male) and hope (female), despair and miracles, a child wasting away and a child blossoming. These opposites, moreover, are reconciled within a framework that is in itself a hybrid—the alternative medicine, hospital-affiliated clinic.

The story then moves from the patient to the practitioner, emphasizing his background in conventional medicine. "Twice a week, after finishing his day's work at the children's department in the hospital, Dr P. undergoes a 'switch' and moves over to the unit in Chinese medicine at the NCM clinic." The story's emphasis moves to the MD's ongoing affiliation with the conventional establishment, the fact that the clinic is "part of the hospital," and the use of conventional methods of diagnosis such as X rays and blood tests. All this establishes a familiar, respectable backdrop for the introduction of the counterclaims of alternative medicine and its implicit criticism of the practices of conventional medicine. Dr. P. does not like to "throw antibiotics around." Describing biomedical work, P. says: "The sick fund doctor sees 30 to 40 children a day. From a technical point of view he cannot tell them all to come back the next day for reevaluation, and he has to make sure that in the event of a sickness developing, the child is covered." Then comes reconciliation. The "alternative" becomes "complementary" as alternative medicine positions itself not in opposition to, but alongside the dominant mainstream. Dr. P. does not rule out the use of antibiotics when necessary, yet

> so long as patients are in a condition in which holding back conventional treatment does not endanger them, I can try and treat them with alternative methods. When one succeeds in overcoming an allergy by means of dietary variation, homeopathy or acupuncture instead of antihistamines—the gain is enormous. Forgetting that the body has the capacity to heal itself, one inundates it with a million medications.

The story then moves on to Dr. R., who is as a general practitioner and a homeopath. Dr. R.'s philosophy serves to extend the medical gaze by addressing the issue of etiology, causality, and cure according to homeopathic theory. Homeopathic medication, according to R.,

> activates the body's healing power and therefore the improvement or cure are real not artificial. . . . Conversely, an antibiotic only kills the germ. Although the inflammation is curtailed, the root of the problem remains untreated, causing recurrent inflammations. To our dismay, a child who is treated with antibiotics four or five times a year due to throat or ear infections is not considered a sickly child, despite the fact that, in our opinion, this indicates something wrong with the body's

resistance. Action taken, such as removing the tonsils or adenoids, is not the correct solution in the majority of cases. The recurrent throat infections will stop, but due to the fact that the source of the problem has not been treated, the sickness will return at a later stage, possibly in other systems of the body, usually more important internal organs. The result can be asthma, arthritis and even behavioral problems. The real solution must contend with the internal reason, which is behind the throat infections. And that is what the homeopathic cure does. That is why its cure is real.

Dr. R., like many other NCM practitioners, is redefining the concept of cure, describing cure reached by conventional means as a non-cure, while introducing concepts such as "superficial" as opposed to "deep."

From these two interviews it is apparent that although the MDs practicing NCM do much to undermine conventional medical treatment, they do not take an exclusively antiestablishment stand. In the closing paragraph of the article, Dr. P. states:

It is not conventional medicine as opposed to alternative medicine... but combined medicine. Integration and maximal use of all methods available in conventional and nonconventional medicine for the benefit of the patient. Under no circumstances do I rule out conventional medicine. I'm just trying to change the structure of the pyramid. It is preferable to start out with the nonconventional methods because they have fewer side effects. When one is not helped by complementary medicine, one can move on to conventional treatment.

This message, albeit delivered with all due respect to conventional medicine, is also revolutionary. It involves direct communication with the public, implicitly undermining the status of conventional medicine, and shaking public confidence in conventional treatments. This is achieved by pointing out the potential harm involved in conventional medicines such as antibiotics and antihistamines, redefining the concept of cure into "real" and "pseudo," and suggesting a radical change in the structure and priorities of medical care. Taking advantage of the authoritative status of conventional medicine (the fact that both interviewees are MDs is emphasized), the status of this medicine is undermined from within.

The article ends with a frame containing advice for administering nonconventional first aid at home. Titled "Don't lower a fever," this frame is particularly interesting as the advice contained there seemingly empowers the parent to deal with minor ailments with simple, "natural" means, "freeing" the person from dependence on conventional medicine.

Story 2: Food Causes Depression

In the Hebrew original this is a play on the adage that "tasty food causes a healthy appetite." This story (*Yediot* 7.16.1993) describes the therapeutic aspects of the food we do or do not eat, ascribing the familiar (food) with a perilous aspect. In this manner, the so-called liberating properties of NCM paradoxically medicalize everyday life. A number of narratives unfold the stories of individuals who were either overstimulated and unable to sit still for a moment, or sleepy, sluggish, and depressed. These problems were solved in a matter of days or weeks by changes in their diets. The theoretical support for the therapeutic potential of diet/nutrition is drawn from ancient medicine—in fact from the father of conventional medicine: "Medicine has always been aware of the value of food in healing—'let your food be your medication, and your medication be your food' was what Hippocrates, the father of medicine, taught his students 2,500 years ago." The reader is then informed that, until the beginning of the twentieth century, ancient theories of nutrition served as the basis for treatment, drawing on the philosophical concept of "a healthy mind in a healthy body." In the twentieth century, unfortunately, thousands of years of experience have been abandoned because "Medicine has moved into the laboratory and become less clinical, and more biological and technical. Only in the last 20 years has there been a return to the idea that nutrition can constitute a component in the treatment not only of depression . . . but of a number of other serious or slight disturbances."

To illustrate this point two stories follow, recounting the respite from symptoms of schizophrenia and combat shock due to changes in diet. The nutritionist interviewed claims that control of the psyche via dietary regulation is not commonly accepted by psychiatrists who are intent on defending their professional prerogative and preventing the entry of other health disciplines. This stand is described as surprising due to the fact that psychiatrists routinely prescribe medication for mental conditions based on the assumption of a connection between chemical imbalance and mental illness. These same psychiatrists are, however, unwilling to admit the causal relationship between foodstuffs and chemical imbalance.

The nutritionist also discusses the pertinence of nutrition to general, mental well-being.

> Events that can happen to anybody—a son being drafted, divorce or bereavement—all take a heavy mental and physical toll. And just then, the inclination is to avoid eating . . . and that upsets the balance even more, because without food, our brain is too weak to think logically, and our nerves are too strung out to take the tension. In my opinion, any person in the process of getting a divorce, any child whose parents are getting divorced, should eat more wholesome food than before. . . . Any person who feels a change in their mood should check what they are eating. Sometimes people say to me "but I always ate like that and I felt all right." True, but perhaps for their new psychological needs, this is not enough anymore.

This connection between mood and food extends the realm traditionally covered by nutrition. In the public view, nutrition has been viewed as a way to maintain physical health, or, as the proverb goes, an apple a day keeps the doctor away. Dr. S., the nutritionist, sums it up by saying:

> If a person feels well and functions well, they can carry on eating as they always have. However, if someone has a problem or wants to maximize their functioning, it is worthwhile going for a single consultation, somewhat like reading a compass. People consult accountants or lawyers in order to manage their financial affairs better. Dietary consultation is a means to better management of the body and mind.

It is interesting to note that the focus of the article is not on physiology—control of cholesterol or blood pressure by means of nutrition—but on control of the psyche. This constitutes a direct extension of the medical gaze. Everyday life is being controlled by experts, control that has now extended from the physical to the more elusive realm of the psyche.

Story 3: Will Power

While the first article focused on MDs, and the second on an academic, paramedical practitioner (a clinical dietician with a PhD), the third article examines the powers of a healer who works through energy transfer and telepathy. This story is therefore the most problematic from a "rational" point of view.

The story (*Yediot* 5.5.1993) of V., a telepathic healer ("he can—but won't—bend spoons"), described the "almost impossible connection" between a person with inexplicable powers and a hospital unit. V. discussed the need for a professional association that would control the activities of healers claiming to have supernatural powers. He personally claims to have subordinated his abilities to the diagnostic constructs of the medical profession, stating that he would never treat a patient who approaches him as a first resort—all patients are initially referred to conventional medicine for evaluation.

> I don't feel as if I am competing with conventional medicine. On the contrary, if they can help—why not? When I am sick, I go to the doctor first and take antibiotics. But one has to acknowledge the fact that medicine has its limits. Sometimes people are so full of medication that it just doesn't effect them anymore, and sometimes there are terrible side effects. Sometimes doctors know how to treat the symptoms, but not the problem itself, and sometimes they are simply helpless.

Once again, conventional medicine is awarded due respect, and then its limitations discussed. The article then introduces Dr. D., a physician who explains that his philosophy is to enable patients to receive nonconventional treatments under conventional medical supervision. Dr. D. first met V. on a television program, was impressed, and sent him a patient. V. helped the patient and, after Dr. D. had met a number of other patients who were being treated by V. at the time, he "was convinced that the 'magic' was worth a try." In reply to the journalist's question whether he had difficulty in accepting V.'s method of treatment, Dr. D. countered that he "didn't have to understand something in order to see it working. Perhaps in ten years we will understand. From my point of view, if the patients feel that V. is helping them, and if I am convinced that it is harmless, I have no problem with it at all. In the year 400 B.C. Hippocrates made a very important statement: 'A doctor has one purpose: to heal!'"

Deus ex Machina—Biomedicine as the Organizing Principle

These three stories are quite typical in their descriptions of the professional strategies of NCM practitioners. Whereas conventional medicine is subjected to criticism, it still provides the authoritative framework for legitimizing and validating NCM modalities. These expositions therefore bring to mind the ancient practice of ending stage plays by having a player in the role of God provide the denouement after being lowered onto the stage by a crane ("deus ex machina"). This player organized the events, conveyed a sense of order to spectators, and pointed out the inevitable or unavoidable design of things. It would appear that in these three stories, the ever-present "deus" seems to be that of conventional medicine, even though it is undermined and criticized, either explicitly or implicitly. Scientific proof and chemistry retain their status as encompassing criteria, and the father of medicine, Hippocrates, is evoked and appropriated by alternative practitioners. This seems to indicate not a split, but a strategy based on reinterpretation of medicine "as it should be." NCM claims to be the true perpetuator of the original Hippocratic philosophy and practice that provided the original premises for biomedical culture before biomedicine strayed into a mechanical and reductionist worldview. This narrative does not indicate wholesale rejection of conventional medical practice but introduces the issue of a more "authentic" interpretation of Hippocrates. This narrative also serves, however, to stress the shared historic source of CM and NCM—creating common grounds and dialogue rather than rejection and exclusion.

NCM's unique contribution to human physical and psychological well-being rests, according to these stories, on the extension of the conventional medical gaze that concentrates mainly on the material. NCM offers a complementary "hearing" (as opposed to the mechanical, intrusive "gaze") that may, however, also result in a greater medicalization of society. This is evident in the definition of cure as "pseudo" versus "real," or "superficial" as opposed to "deep." This perception contends that lack of symptoms does not necessarily mean that a person is healthy. Consequently, NCM goes well beyond what is offered by conventional medicine in terms of treatment and also in terms of control. The body's self-healing capacity, alluded to so often in alternative medicine, does not change the body from object to subject, but further objectifies the body. The body is not "set free" by the NCM presented in these stories, but is further ensnared by an additional set of experts on the rise.

The symbols evoked in these stories constitute an interesting fusion of opposites. Dr. P. crosses the border every day, moving from the hospital department to the complementary clinic. The clinic, however, is not represented as extraterritorial. The presence of various MDs in the clinic, and its location on hospital grounds, constitute a fusion of the familiar and the foreign. This indicates successful domestication, representing high acculturation to biomedicine as well as high assimilation—measured in acceptance both by the establishment and the public. Such domestication is evident in Dr. P's ideology, which refuses to choose between alternative and conventional, opting instead for what he calls "combined medicine."

These three tales of NCM also suggest a new way of looking at the body. The scope of medical care is extended to include a fusion between body and mind, creating what has come to be known as the "holistic approach." NCM ideology often focuses on stimulating the body's own potential for self-healing, thereby turning the patient into a partner. However, this notion of self-help contains a paradox because it relies on a new class of experts—NCM practitioners—for its realization. More control is therefore gained in the name of partnership. This is what I call the paradox of empowerment and objectification. The message of empowerment, taken on its own, would seem completely revolutionary in the field of health care. However, closer scrutiny has shown that the popular discourse of NCM in fact reframes the notion of empowerment, introducing new experts who control new entities, thereby effectively extending the scope of dependence and, indeed, medicalization.

Conventional Medicine Fights Back

Many of the more positive stories on NCM in the media show how people who had lost hope and faith in conventional medicine were miraculously saved by NCM. These stories are countered by representatives of CM who make use of the media to warn the public about the dangers of seemingly "natural" products and practitioners who are not properly qualified. These two narrative categories represent, respectively, "magic moments" and "horror stories." The "horror stories" do not deny the popularity and success of NCM. Indeed, it is the popularity of NCM that renders it especially hazardous in this context. The horror stories portray the dark side of NCM, depicting it as irresponsible and deleterious. In contrast, the "magic moments" category emphasizes the bright and, indeed, miraculous side of NCM, and the benefits inherent in its alternative lifestyle and worldview.

As the borders of conventional medicine are manipulated by NCM practitioners who attempt at once to criticize conventional medicine while pointing out its shared characteristics with NCM, CM practitioners engage in similar strategies. However, this time, it is NCM that is criticized as dangerous and potentially harmful, especially when not practiced under the supervision of MDs. In this manner the "magic moments" and "miraculous cures" described in articles on NCM are dampened by warnings and "horror stories" that present the danger inherent in unsupervised NCM treatment. These stories do not deny the popularity and success of NCM. Indeed it is this very popularity that calls for the intervention of conventional medicine in order to tame, indeed domesticate, the errant discipline. It is interesting to note that both the narratives of CM and NCM sustain the authority of biomedicine, although there might be some argument about its hegemony on the part of NCM practitioners who suggest "inverting the pyramid" or integrating the two types of medicine into a new "combined medicine."

Horror Stories

A recent article on NCM products (*The Jerusalem Post* 9. 9. 2001) began in a chilling tone:

> They sit innocently on the shelves of pharmacies and health food stores, and you can pick them up and pay at the cash register without asking—or being asked—any questions. More Israelis than ever are buying herbal supplements in the hope that they will relieve, or even cure, conditions ranging from allergies to psychiatric problems. Many physicians tended to ignore these pills and powders, dismissing them as offering a mere placebo effect, if any at all. But with such widespread use doctors are being forced to pay attention.

The dire consequences of unsupervised use of NCM is a recurrent theme in the communication of conventional doctors with the public.

For example, the problem of self-medication with 'natural' over-the-counter drugs is discussed by a prominent neurologist (*Yediot* 18.2.2000) who tells of patients suffering from epilepsy who had fits because they had taken a 'natural' product containing zinc, which is forbidden to epileptic patients. Another professor who specializes in hypertension describes patients whose balance of fluids had been upset due to unwise use of NCM: "We see patients who have high blood pressure, whose legs are swollen, and when we ask them they tell us that they are taking a medication that has licorice extract in it. This is harmful to them. There are a large number of preparations that affect the balance of fluids in the body or the absorption of salt. We have also seen kidney damage due to mistaken use of natural remedies."

An article entitled "Natural is not always healthy" (*Haaretz* 5.3.2000) also concentrates on the potential damage inherent in unsupervised use of herbal remedies. A professor of neurology summarizes the situation: "Herbal products should be dealt with in the same manner as conventional medications. They should not be prescribed for an individual who has not been examined and they should not be given for certain symptoms until one knows what causes them. First of all one has to be diagnosed by a doctor and only then can one know what it is permissible to take." A specialist in allergies describes two patients whom he sent to NCM practitioners as part of an "experiment." They were misdiagnosed and the treatment recommended could have endangered them. The potentially dangerous effects of gingko on pregnant women and their fetuses are described in another article (*The Jerusalem Post* 9.9. 2001) and a conventional physician interviewed in the article suggests that "patients should be questioned about their use of herbal supplements in a nonjudgmental way, and the information retained in their files." Summing up the situation, the deputy director of the Ministry of Health is quoted as saying that: "a system of supervision will have to be established in order to regulate this field which is unsupervised."

In the same manner that NCM practitioners recommend NCM as a manner of avoiding the perils of biomedicine, such as negative side effects of antibiotics, conventional doctors are recommending biomedical supervision of NCM as a way of avoiding the potential dangers of NCM. It is, however, interesting to note a certain paradox. NCM is presented as potentially harmful, whereas it is also portrayed as impotent, ineffective, and a "waste of time." This claim usually goes hand in hand with claims of the relationship between science and biomedicine. In an article on migraines (*Maariv* 3.5.2000) a prominent neurologist states: "In most of the clinics across the world where migraines are treated, alternative medicine is not used because it is less effective. The alternative approach is problematic because research that uses scientific criteria to examine the efficacy of treatments such as acupuncture, reflexology, homeopathy or herbs does not exist. We did a study on the efficiency of a certain herbal remedy and found it less effective than a placebo."

In an article on spastic bronchitis among children, a pediatrician states that nonconventional therapies are "treatments that are unscientific and unproven whereas medical treatments can offer a solution which has been clinically tested" (*Maariv* 10.1.2000). Discussing CFS, another MD describes the problems involved in treating the syndrome. The opinion expressed is that "NCM does not have a cure that is suitable for everyone and only a few people have been cured by NCM treatments. There are also charlatans who take advantage of the patient's situation and can in certain cases even cause damage."

Conventional medicine therefore portrays itself to the public as qualified to protect it from the potential dangers of NCM, or conversely, from wasting time due to the inefficacy of many of the modalities. The need to supervise NCM treatments is then extended to the necessity of protecting patients from NCM practitioners who are often portrayed as charlatans or abusive. NCM users are described as being psychologically vulnerable and therefore all the more in need of protection by the medical establishment. In an article published in *The Jerusalem Post* (13.5. 2000) a university psychologist states that "unbalanced people who go to complementary practitioners may get into trouble.... People who have emotional problems or have undergone trauma who voluntarily go to complementary practitioners don't know what to expect, and after the treatment may find their condition has worsened." Referring to a case in which an alternative practitioner had been accused of sexually abusing his female client, the article suggested that NCM practitioners should be barred from touching their patients, unless the place to be touched has been identified in advance and the patient has expressed consent after receiving a full explanation. The possibility of sexual abuse is thus connected to "touch," which has become a symbol of NCM. A connection is thus constructed between NCM and sexual abuse, thereby adding another dimension to the need for supervision.

In these stories, conventional doctors are in fact countering the therapeutic claims made by NCM practitioners. On the one hand these NCM modalities are described as dangerous and potent. When not used properly, they have the capacity to cause real damage. However, on the other hand these same modalities are described as impotent and at times even less effective than a placebo. This might be an attempt to dampen the public's enthusiasm for NCM treatments. However, the point is clearly made that all NCM treatment should be conducted under medical supervision. In this manner the medical profession is reasserting, this time on the pages of the daily press, its claim for hegemony in the treatment of patients, the diagnosis of disease, and the prescription of medicines of any sort. As we have seen, the NCM practitioners interviewed do not explicitly suggest abandoning conventional medicine, but rather are in the process of seeking ways to integrate the two approaches. This search for integration could serve as one of the major forces behind the domestication of NCM. Biomedical authority is not attacked in the dissemination of NCM to the public by NCM practitioners. Whenever possible, the authority of biomedicine is called on to prove NCM claims, and NCM practitioners who are also conventional MDs make use of this fact to validate their claims for the benefits of NCM. What does seem to be under attack, however, is the hegemony of biomedicine. NCM practitioners suggest integration of both methods or even "reversing the structure of the pyramid"—that is, first trying NCM modalities and, when these are unsuccessful, resorting to biomedicine. This implies a pluralistic approach to health care, which, at the end of the day, is most probably not acceptable to the medical establishment. The medical establishment in charge of health services and policy-making retains the power to decide to what extent, on what terms, and indeed, if at all, NCM practice will be allowed (Fadlon et al., 2003).

This state of affairs is particularly well illustrated in an article (*Maariv* 10.12.1997) "There is an alternative" that describes the hospital-adjacent NCM clinics in Israel and their relationship with the hospital and its staff. The (non-MD) director of one hospital clinic recounts a situation in which "there still are doctors who find it hard to accept us and I can understand them. A doctor who has put so many years into his training has to face practitioners who have only studied for a few years and use simple means of diagnosis. One should remember that NCM is only complementary medicine and does not assume to take the place of conventional medicine." At another hospital, the clinic director (a non-MD, NCM practitioner) describes a situation in which "We are welcome in the hospital departments and the contact with the doctors is positive but not sufficient." He objects to the distinction between CM and NCM and says: "There is one medicine—that which helps patients. We hope to achieve a situation similar to that in China where both modalities are integrated. We are on the right track. We have reached the stage where patients are tired of using pain killers and antibiotics." Yet another clinic director describes a situation in which patients are referred to the clinic, but not much clinical cooperation exists with the hospital wards. "Some of our patients approach the clinic independently and others are referred through doctors at the hospital. We are hoping that in the future there will be full cooperation with the hospital wards and that we will be able to serve an advisory capacity in the hospital wards."

Although it is clear from the description of the interaction between the clinics and the hospital wards that the nature, extent, and intensity of such cooperation depends on the goodwill of the conventional MDs at the hospital, the NCM practitioners view such cooperation and integration as an important goal. Nonetheless, the very existence of these clinics contributes much to the legitimation of NCM in the public eye by stressing the commitment to cooperation with biomedicine. In this process, NCM forgoes many of its exotic claims and basic philosophy, thus becoming domesticated into the dominant ideology of biomedicine.

Chapter 6

Institutionalization: The NCM College

The Flexner report constituted a turning point in the professionalization of American medicine. Prior to that report, a large number of medical schools flourished and, in the absence of any external (professional or educational) control, these schools offered medical degrees as part of a profit-making venture (Cockerham, 1986). Students were admitted on the basis of their ability to pay admission and tuition fees, which ultimately resulted in low- quality medical education as well as low prestige for physicians. In 1904 the AMA (American Medical Association) established the Council on Medical Education in order to consolidate suggestions for the improvement of education. The council subsequently attained the status of a regulatory agency, thereby strengthening the influence of the AMA in medical education. With its publication in 1910, the Flexner Report provided an overall evaluation of the standard of medical education throughout the United States, and proposed guidelines for the establishment of a uniform course of studies as well as facilities necessary for the education of physicians. In this manner, the basis for cooperation between the state and the medical profession was consolidated. The medical profession was thus instrumental in creating uniformity in the content of medical education and gained control over the licensing of university graduates as physicians.

Medical schools provide the site for education and socialization of the MD. This process has been recently studied by Good (1994), who focused on how the American medical student comes to view the human body. Shuval (1980), in a study conducted in Israel, pointed out a unique orga-

---

Pseudonyms are used throughout this chapter.

nizational aspect of medical education. In Israel, clinical tutors also serve as potential employers because practicing private medicine is not generally a full-time option. This dual role of mentor–employer enhances conformity.

The professionalization of medicine in the United States, which culminated in the control and regulation of medical education by the medical profession, was initiated by a core of American physicians educated in Europe. These physicians formed an association that was powerful enough to set the standards for all medical education. When examining the institutions that teach NCM in Israel, we find an equally interesting situation that brings to mind medical education in the United States prior to the Flexner Report. This situation is characterized by lack of uniformity and collective guidelines. No formal relationship has yet been established between practitioners of NCM and the state and therefore a common curriculum does not exist. The alternative therapist is thus the product of an institution that is not formally under the supervision of the medical establishment, even though training culminates in therapeutic practice.

Israeli law prohibits the treatment of patients by individuals who have no formal medical training. There is therefore no uniform course of studies for the alternative practitioner, obviously no state examination (as in nursing or medicine), and no formal licensing process. This situation has led the larger institutions that currently operate in the field to establish agreements with American and Chinese institutions of learning that oversee the academic program and in some cases provide a diploma. The Israeli colleges therefore maintain ties with representatives from the East (China) and the West (America). These ties can be viewed as providing some sort of academic framework and they compensate for the absence of local guidelines. The Israeli Council of Higher Education does not recognize the diplomas granted by these foreign institutions for two reasons:

1. The right to practice medicine is limited to licensed MDs, with certain concessions made to paramedical professions such as nursing, physiotherapy, and lately also chiropracters. A foreign diploma bearing witness to capabilities in NCM does not therefore render practice within the Israeli context legal.

2. Licensed MDs are permitted to use any method of treatment that they perceive to be beneficial to the patient, providing in-

formed consent has been given. The MD's command of one alternative therapy or another is not an issue that is under legal or professional scrutiny.

Although NCM colleges have claimed that formal recognition for their program in Israel is "just around the corner," such recognition has not yet been granted. However, the anticipation of recognition and its prerequisites has probably had some bearing on the curricula of these colleges and created a unique intellectual climate.

The dilemmas encountered by different institutions for the teaching of NCM seem quite similar. Baer et al. (1998) and Cant and Sharma (1996) have studied such institutions in the San Francisco Bay Area and in England, respectively. In a study conducted on a college teaching acupuncture in the San Francisco Bay Area, Baer (1998) discussed two dimensions of professionalization: (1) the very establishment of these schools, and (2) the acculturation to the biomedical model in the teaching of NCM. Baer points out that students are required to spend a considerable amount of time studying courses in Western sciences. Along with this acculturation to biomedicine, professional behavior is also formulated in the image of biomedical symbolism. Quoting from the yearbook of one institution, which teaches acupuncture, Baer described the required appearance for students: "Students should be professionals in both appearance and attitude, being neat and clean at all times. White lab coats with a name tag appropriately identifying the students as Observer, Trainee I, Trainee II or Intern are required" (1998: 535).

Cant and Sharma (1996), who studied a number of nonmedical colleges that were engaged in the instruction of homeopathy in England, have pointed out that although no harmonization of standards existed, nonmedical homeopathy has realized that reference to the biomedical model is imperative. One practitioner interviewed admitted that "we have to interpret homeopathy according to our modern understandings. I prefer to talk about homeostasis rather than the vital force, the meta-matter understanding is inappropriate" (1996: 583). Another instructor at one such institution commented: "We have to teach a very specific pathological type of homeopathy, which is not the best way of doing things." In the curricula of these colleges the more controversial teachings and esoteric elements have been deemphasized and the colleges have gradually recruited state-registered nurses and MDs to teach anatomy and physiology, thus adopting mainstream medical teachings.

In general, the professionalization project of homeopathy has been associated with the development of "scientific knowledge" within the discipline. There has been a consistent effort to attach homeopathy to the scientific paradigm and hope has been expressed that in the future "bio-physics will offer an explanation" (1996: 585), and that homeopathy will be able to enlist science to prove that, in practice, its therapy works.

Cant and Sharma (1996) also illustrated the manner in which practitioners make efforts to package themselves as mainstream and not marginal. One practitioner described the process in the following manner: "We used to be a bunch of old Hippies practising away in our front rooms; it was a cottage industry, now we are professionals and we have to act, and I am afraid, even dress like professionals. I used to have hair down to my shoulders, smoke dope—but we have evolved" (1996: 585).

As we will see, similar elements to those described in the United States and England exist in the teaching of NCM in the Israeli colleges. I would, however, like to point out that the effort to domesticate NCM also involves the construction of new, hybrid symbols.

Applicants can get to know their institute of choice through introductory lectures that are open to the general public. These lectures usually lay out the principles of NCM, principles of practice within Israeli law, and procedures of study, training, and internship (here the "trip to the Chinese affiliate" figures prominently). Written material is available to potential students in the form of the college yearbook. These booklets contain information on the various courses in the curriculum and give a sense of the outlook embraced by the college. Once enrolled, the student participates in a unique process: the dissemination of non-Western, noncontemporary, nonconventional theories of healing that have been transferred to a Western context. The particular mixture of biomedicine and NCM therapies is managed by each school on an individual basis. This is also a case of domestication in action. I will demonstrate this process by examining the content of introductory lectures, yearbooks, and the quarterly college bulletin.

Introductory Lecture for Potential Students

This lecture was basically open to the general public with the intention of appealing to potential students. The meeting lasted for five hours, and started with a tour of the school's clinic. In the course of the tour, emphasis was placed on the professional, practical aspect of the course of studies. In a taken-for-granted manner it was promised that studies would lead to employment. The feeling was that the participants were not only potential students, but also potential lessors of the clinic's premises. The dean of the college showed us around the rooms, pointing out examination couches, the wall-to-wall carpeting, and the fact that each room had running water. Proceeding upstairs to the lecture room, we passed through the lobby of the college, an area that was both "Oriental" and "medical." The walls were decorated with Oriental anatomical charts that showed meridians and acupuncture points and other symbols of the Far East, such as an oversized parchment fan often used in the decoration of Chinese restaurants. At another college, the walls in the lobby were lined with glass cabinets filled with crystals, Chinese medicine apparatus such as moxa, acupuncture needles, and thick glass bottles labeled with Chinese lettering. Adjacent to these cabinets was a board on which students' grades had been posted.

The lecture itself concentrated less on philosophy than on actual practice, once again strengthening the "hands-on" approach created during the tour. This could indeed be viewed as an attempt to play down the more esoteric parts of NCM at this stage by avoiding the issue altogether. The owner of the college, who has a background in NCM and assumed the title "dean," discussed the difference between Oriental and Western medicine. A new etiology of illness was introduced by means of concepts such as system imbalance and impaired flow of energy. These causes of sickness were accessible through diagnostic methods unknown in the West, such as measuring the pulse or surveying the tongue. The forty-odd people sitting in the room were then asked to stick out their tongues and the dean moved from one to the next, inspecting while making humming and hawing sounds. Some tongues were approved "all right," and remarks were ventured about others. Passing by a young woman in the back row, he remarked: "Oh, you're having a period, aren't you?" and, without waiting for her response, moved on. The woman nodded animatedly at the young man sitting beside her, an expression of amazement spreading across her face.

A volunteer was then called up. After some reluctance, a young man agreed to cooperate. Stripped of his shirt, his belt unbuckled and trouser button open, the young man lay on his stomach on a medical examination table with his arms stretched out in front. An Israeli expert in Chinese medicine, who had joined us, proceeded to examine his back. The expert, called Tommy, was introduced by the dean as someone who had a lot of energy to give. This was explained using the Chinese concept of yin-yang. Students were warned that "giving" too much energy in treatment would tax them and they were advised not to work beyond their limits. Tommy was described as an individual with exceptional "giving" capacity, which enabled him to perform a large number of treatments. Tommy, balding, with a long plait and Chinese-style goatee smiled at us and tugged at the young man's trousers to gain access to the lower back, exposing his buttocks. The young man grinned in embarrassment and tried to pull his pants up again. Both the dean and Tommy reassured him; this was anatomy, we were all colleagues, and this is how we learned about the body—observing, touching, manipulating.

The expert then asked the volunteer a number of questions. The young man turned over to lie on his back, seemingly at ease, this time almost parodying his partial nakedness by overemphasizing his efforts to readjust his trousers. The acupuncture point was selected and disinfected and an acupuncture needle, which seemed to be at least 7 cm long, was plunged into his epigastrium. This demonstration of skill, inserting a somewhat long needle into an area near the heart, was appreciated by the audience and displayed a level of expertise to which potential students could aspire.

Using the human body to demonstrate diagnostic and therapeutic skill is generally the exclusive prerogative of the medical profession. The demonstration of diagnosis and therapy in the introductory lecture had appropriated practices of the medical school, claiming this prerogative for alternative medicine as well. A similar performative fusion of NCM and biomedicine was also adopted by Dr. N. (the MD in charge of a hospital-adjacent NCM clinic) at a seminar for clinical nursing tutors. Dr. N. created common (conventional) grounds with his audience by basing much of his lecture on biological facts. He cited the "well-known" fact that 80 to 90% of the population can spontaneously recover even from infection by the most pathogenic germ. Despite this fact, conventional medicine is based on dependence on external methods, tending to forget the body's own powers of healing. One of the body's methods of self-healing is running a temperature. Conventional medicine tends to lower the temperature instead of letting the body do its work.

The following exchange then took place with a member of the audience.

Q. According to the approach you presented, when a person has a temperature of 38.5° Celsius, paracetamol shouldn't be given. The temperature might then climb to 40° C.

A. In your career, how many patients have you seen with a temperature of 40° C?

Q. My children.

A. 40° C is not a tragedy. You know, let's talk chemistry. I'm pleased you brought this up. When can biological damage occur? At 41° C. What I'm saying is that the limit should be raised. Medication is given for a high temperature in order to prevent damage. A biological reaction will only occur at 41° C, 42° C. If we exclude the population with a tendency for convulsions, one can indeed let a temperature rise in a controlled manner. This does indeed call for a greater effort in observing the patient instead of saying "now I'll have four hours of peace and quiet." Observation and monitoring of existing mechanisms in the body are very important. If you can't watch a child, then you medicate.

Q. You're not dealing with the child's discomfort—don't you want to alleviate that?

A. Alternative medicine has ways and means of alleviating suffering during an illness by prescribing additional methods. This is not the time and place to describe them. The question is whether to gain the marked advantage of a high temperature. A high temperature is the result of a positive process. One has to decide: to hell with the process, just let's get rid of the temperature or go along with the process.

In the course of this lecture, Dr. N. took advantage of scientific discourse to prove a point in alternative medicine. Conventional medicine was described as the easy, unnatural resort.

The Yearbook

The graphics and logo of the yearbooks evoke a sense of Orientalism (Said, 1993). The front page of one book is decorated with a male silhouette in blue with white acupuncture points dotting the body, which is encompassed by an arrow, evoking the idea of a holistic embrace. The cover of another yearbook employs a colorful fourfold representation of the ying-yang symbol that is duplicated on the top of every page. The inside cover bears an ancient Chinese quote that appears three times, in English, in Hebrew, and in Chinese calligraphy:

> *In peaceful calm,*
> *Void and emptiness,*
> *The authentic qi*
> *Flows easily.*
> *Essences and spirits*
> *Are kept within.*
> *How could illnesses arise?*

This quote encapsulates the philosophy of Chinese medicine that illness is due to blockage of the flow of energies. The "peaceful calm" also appears to be an antithesis to the jumpy and crowded postmodern world that we inhabit.

The yearbooks also contain a message to students from the dean of the college. This message appears at the beginning of the yearbook and is accompanied by a photograph of the dean sitting at his desk in a suit and tie, a weighty volume to his left and his hand resting on an open ledger. The very existence of the position of "dean"—an academic position belonging to the Western, academic world—indicates the Western framework within which the "other" will be taught. The message, in full, reads as follows:

Dear Student,

Relating to the need to **eradicate the cause of sickness and not only the symptoms thereof**, in accordance with the wish to treat the person as a whole, we have chosen to establish **an institution in which we will offer instruction in the medicine of the 21st century—the art and science of natural-**complementary **medicine.**

Due to instinctive wisdom and realization of the inner value of the arts of natural healing, many of the citizens of Israel have opted for the incorporation of natural medicine within the framework of existing health services.

At present, complementary medicine is joining forces with conventional medicine and in addition to the many private clinics for complementary medicine which already exist, clinics offering treatments in acupuncture, homeopathy and complementary medicine have been established in hospitals. Also some of the sick funds provide the option for treatment by methods belonging to complementary medicine.

We have therefore anticipated the need to establish the infrastructure for a health care system, which perceives of the body and spirit as one unit. We have anticipated the need to **establish a generation of healers who are not just technicians**.

We recognize the fact that various cultures in the past and present have much to offer us. Our purpose and aspiration at Nature's Complementary College is to combine the wisdom and the harmony of oriental medicine and naturopathy with the innovations of modern medicine and society.

The course of studies in the four year programs are at an academic level and the professional programs are conducted by means of knowledge agreements and professional supervision of leading colleges in Europe and America.

By means of research and a high standard of teaching we will acquire a better understanding of the situation of mankind.

We, the directors and teachers at Nature's Complementary College, are well aware of the importance of co-operation between natural, complementary medicine and modern medicine and address the challenge of providing suitable professional training.

Nature's Complementary College was established 15 years ago and is the largest and oldest institution in Israel for studies and professional training in the field of complementary medicine, with subsidiaries in Tel Aviv, Haifa and Jerusalem.

The various subsidiaries are situated in the city center and are easily reached. The main subsidiary in Tel Aviv includes a sophisticated clinic and a large library and is situated nearby the central station.

If you would like to be at the forefront of a new, interesting and sought-after profession, and at the same time experience the tradition of natural medicine which is thousands of years old—join us, and come to learn at Nature's Complementary College.

The dean's message describes the college as a hypermodern institution, which teaches "the medicine of the twenty-first century"—a medicine that is a hybrid construct, comprising "the art and science of natural, complementary medicine." The college subscribes to the fact that "different cultures, past and present, have much to offer us" and therefore aspires to "incorporate the wisdom and harmony of oriental medicine and naturopathy with the innovations of modern society and medicine."

Students are invited to join the college if they want to be "at the forefront of a new, interesting and sought-after profession and experience at the same time the tradition of natural medicine, which is thousands of years old." Although the medical profession is implicitly criticized through the dean's wish to "create a generation of healers, who are not just technicians," on the whole the college does not adopt an antiestablishment stand. The impression is that of cooperation between the medical establishment and the "complementary natural medicine" taught at the college.

The college offers two main programs of "academic level" courses (which are not recognized by the Israeli medical establishment or any other state licensing body such as the council for higher education). These programs are presented in the yearbook as "The Faculty for Chinese Medicine" and "The Faculty for Naturopathy."

The Oriental Medicine Curriculum

The four-year curriculum in Chinese medicine is divided into five main tracks: (1) courses in Chinese medicine, (2) Chinese herbology, (3) complementary healing arts, (4) Western sciences, and (5) clinical specialization.

Courses in Chinese Medicine

The following courses constitute this section: clinical Oriental medicine, diagnosis and evaluation, and laboratory for detection of acupuncture points. Noteworthy here is the course in clinical Oriental medicine, which is described as a course that "provides the student with a detailed description of western medical diagnostic techniques for common complaints and illnesses and the corresponding treatments in traditional oriental medicine." In this manner a fusion is formed between the two systems—diagnosis is performed according to Western techniques and treatment is administered according to traditional Oriental medicine. This no doubt contributes to the domestication of Oriental medicine due to the fact that diagnostic categories or syndromes of traditional Oriental medicine (i.e., "the plum stuck in the throat" syndrome mentioned in the chapter on the clinic) seem irrational in terms of Western biology since they are based on an entirely different concept of anatomy. This fusion, then, renders Oriental treatment less exotic and more familiar. Interesting, too, is the group of courses taught as a "laboratory." This space obviously originates from the Western, scientific, and experimental tradition and its incorporation into the teaching of traditional Oriental medicine serves to create a modern Western image for the detection of acupuncture points that have been around for thousands of years. Among the "clinical techniques" taught to students in the laboratory one finds "sterilization according to techniques acceptable in Israel and California," for example.

Chinese Herbology

This unit teaches students to identify medicinal herbs, herbal mixtures, and the therapeutic use of these herbs. Students are taught the use of herbs according to "modern pathologies" and also according to the tradition of Oriental medicine. Noteworthy, once again, is the recourse to classification of symptoms according to Western diagnostic categories. As in the previous unit, this type of categorization deemphasizes the more esoteric aspects of Chinese philosophy of the body and its original etiology of disease and illness.

Complementary Healing Arts

This unit comprises what the college calls "allied arts." Students are taught therapeutic practices that are not incorporated into the courses in Oriental medicine, such as shiatsu, Western herbology, homeopathy, Oriental nutrition practices, and Chinese ethics and philosophy. These practices probably provide the therapist in Oriental Chinese medicine with a basis in methods, which might be useful in practice later on. In the section on complementary healing arts students are also introduced to the practicalities of running a clinic. The curriculum includes courses in how to organize a clinic, keep medical records, information on tax laws, methods of marketing, joining a clinic in the private and public sector, as well as professional liability and insurance.

Western Sciences

In this unit, students are taught courses in medical terminology. The objective is to improve the students' ability to communicate with various persons within the field of medicine by using a "broad and professional vocabulary." This scientific vocabulary includes biochemistry, biology, anatomy, introduction to neuro-orthopedic evaluation, pathophysiology, clinical sciences, physical examination, pharmacology, biophysics, clinical advice, Western nutrition practices, CPR, and first aid. This emphasis on biomedical vocabulary is in line with the programs described by Baer (1998) and Cant and Sharma (1996). In this manner, although no particular guidelines exist for the licensing of practitioners of NCM in Israel, "biomedicalization" of the field anticipates such future recognition. A major force in the professionalization of NCM therefore includes an acculturation process, which combines the language and practices of NCM with those of biomedicine.

Clinical Specialization

In this unit students take one preclinical course and three courses in clinical specialization, in which they observe the treatment of patients at the college's clinic or at clinics affiliated with the various hospitals with which the college has an agreement for cooperation. Theoretical learning therefore culminates in supervised clinical practice, much in the tradition of medical internship. Although I have described the curriculum for Oriental medicine in detail in the framework of this section, I would like to point out that the other four-year track at the college, naturopathy, similarly incorporates the study of nonconventional practices together with biomedical sciences.

Domesticating the Alternative Gaze

As we have seen, studying Oriental medicine includes subjects such as acupuncture, Chinese herbology, Oriental nutrition methods, and Chinese philosophy and ethics. All these subjects share a view of the body in terms of energy. The idea of *qi*—the essential energy that, when blocked, leads to disease—is basic to the perception of health and illness in the tradition of Chinese medicine. Treatment ideally entails the unblocking of the channels in which the *qi* has been obstructed by means of acupuncture needles. Nutrition is also based on spiritual concepts of hot and cold conditions and corresponding hot and cold diets. Obviously, this view extends the boundaries of embodiment beyond what is normally acceptable in the framework of conventional medicine. The notion of energy, however, does not replace the more material, conventional gaze of the body, which is also at the heart of socialization at the NCM college.

Learning this alternative gaze, which is deemphasized when its tenets seem too far-reaching from the point of view of Western rationality, does not entail rejection of the conventional gaze. Indeed, Western concepts and practices are incorporated into the study of Chinese medicine. As I have pointed out, the group of courses presented under the title "laboratory for the detection of acupuncture points" fuses one of the ultimate symbols of modern Western science with ancient skill. Moreover, the unit in Chinese medicine is completed with a course called "clinical oriental medicine" in which students are familiarized with Western medical diagnostic techniques for common complaints and the corresponding treatments in traditional Oriental medicine. The course in Oriental medicine thus culminates in the construction of a medicine that is neither Chinese nor Western, but a combination. The notion of fusing Western diagnosis with Chinese treatment also somewhat neglects the philosophy of Chinese medicine, its etiology of disease, and the manner in which it constructs the body. Using biomedical diagnostic techniques, the student learns to rephrase a complaint with ginger, cinnamon, and salt water standing in for antibiotics.

Under the title "allied arts," students of Chinese medicine are taught shiatsu, Western herbology, Bach flower therapy, homeopathy, Oriental nutrition, Chinese philosophy and ethics, and clinic management. The rationale for studying allied arts is that "a successful clinic in Oriental medicine does not entail the use of acupuncture and Chinese medicinal herbs alone." This justification is particularly interesting in view of the fact that homeopathy, Western herbology, and Bach flower therapy are all methods that originated in Europe. Combining them with Oriental medicine points to an additional aspect of domestication as well as the fusion of different periods, cultures, and philosophies.

The college also sees to it that its students become versed in Western science. Students are taught anatomy, pathophysiology, biochemistry, first aid, and resuscitation. Noteworthy is the course in "medical terminology" in which students study "the etymology of words used in Western, medical terminology and their use in the description of the physiology and pathology of the body." The explicit goal of this course is to "improve the student's ability to communicate with various figures in the medical field through the use of an extensive and professional vocabulary." Students are also taught how to write a medical report, refer patients to conventional specialists, and decipher X rays and laboratory tests.

The curriculum of the college shows that the wish for incorporation into the medical establishment is more pronounced than the wish to be instrumental in its rejection. Conventional medicine and its practitioners constitute a dominant reference group with which the college is intent on communicating. The vocabulary of conventional medicine is named the *professional* vocabulary. The dominance of biomedicine is probably related to two facts: If and when the State finally decides on criteria for licensing non-MD NCM practitioners, these will probably include knowledge of basic principles of conventional medicine and Western science. Colleges have therefore constructed their curricula in anticipation of these future demands. Moreover, many members of the college staff along with other parties who have an economic interest in the colleges are themselves MDs.

The college and other NCM institutes presented an interesting phenomenon in regard to academic titles. All practitioners and teachers at the colleges who were not MDs freely used the title "Dr" awarded to them by institutes of learning abroad. Because these foreign institutes are not recognized by Israeli licensing boards, an individual who has been awarded the title of "Oriental medical doctor" cannot use the title "Dr." in the Israeli context. However, these practitioners insisted on the use of that title both within and outside of the Israeli colleges. This custom seemed at first to suggest the existence of an independent, even alternative social world. I soon realized, however, that the insistence on these titles actually reflected an artificial symmetry that NCM practitioners were keen to induce between their world and that of biomedicine. In the list of faculty members who appeared in the college yearbooks, for example, the names of staff members appeared with a title followed by the relevant letters of accreditation. There was, for example, Dr. Paolo Maradonna (MD) on the list, apparently a doctor of conventional medicine. On the other hand, the name of Dr. Joe Ramb was followed by the letters OMD, PhD, Ac. These letters imply that the bearer of the title is an "Oriental medical doctor" with a PhD in acupuncture. The use of these letters is interesting because they seem to denote a double claim to the title "doctor," first as an Oriental medical doctor, and second as a PhD in acupuncture. It is also interesting to note that the qualifying letters in parentheses are absent from the prescription pads and receipts used by Joe Ramb. The recourse to prescription pads for prescribing nonprescription drugs is also significant as yet another illustration of acculturation.[1]

The distinction between MDs and non-MDs by means of qualifying letters in parentheses was uniform throughout the yearbooks. Although this could serve to differentiate between MDs and non-MDs for the initiated, in practice, both groups insisted on being addressed as "Dr." This emphasizes the high status enjoyed by MDs in Western society and the aspiration of non-MDs to share this status. Desiring that students and patients perceive them as "doctors," practitioners tended to adopt the paraphernalia of Western medical symbolism—donning white coats and writing prescriptions for nonprescription drugs. A situation different to that described at the college prevailed at the NCM clinic. At staff meetings MDs were always referred to by their colleagues as Dr., whereas the other practitioners—even the chiropractors whose relative position was high—were called by their first names even though they were using the title "Dr." (gained at an overseas institution).

The College Bulletin

The quarterly college bulletin, which is distributed among staff and students, is an important device disseminating information to those already involved in the learning process. This bulletin contributes to the socialization and professionalization of the future therapists and is not intended, like the introductory lecture or yearbook, to capture the interest of potential applicants. Similar to media reportage, these bulletins tended to create and then reconcile differentiation between CM and NCM. One such bulletin included an article written by the head of the department of naturopathy, "Are the latest fashions harmful to health?" In this article, the author constructs a dichotomy between Western society, which "emphasizes external appearances without giving a thought to natural imperatives," and "societies that choose a style of dress which maintains the individual's health in everyday life in the long and short term." This glorified other, unnamed yet existing as a contrast to modern Western society, "acts according to the rules of nature and comprehension of mankind, its ways, physiology, behavioral modes and synchronization with nature." Later on, this notion of the glorified other is qualified as "tribes, nations and peoples we tend to call 'primitive.'"

The examples of harmful Western apparel dictated by fashion include tight clothing in general, particularly brassieres and men's underpants, which interfere with the drainage of poisons by the lymphatic system. This point is used to implicate these garments with a high incidence of cancer. Other fashionable items such as sunglasses with small lenses, high-heel and closed shoes, and clothes that expose the body in summer are also blamed. This article actively preaches an "alternative lifestyle" in line with "green," New Age philosophy. It is interesting to note, however, that justification for this lifestyle is drawn from conventional, scientific research findings. Another article by the same author, which appeared in another bulletin under the title "Research update," constituted an interesting combination of the rejection of the maladies of Western society supported by research findings from reputable scientific institutions. These scientific research findings were again used to legitimize a naturalistic point of view.

The article "Research update" dealt with the connection between stress, television, and heart disease; the beneficial effect of gardens and trees on aggressive behavior; prevention of cataracts by nutrition; and the connection between a certain spice and the prevention of colon cancer, to name a few subjects. Each item is preceded by information concerning the source of the data, such as "a group of researchers from the medical center at Duke University"; "4,730 women participated in an extensive study"; "sounds peculiar? but these are the findings of research by doctors who provide statistical evidence that..."; or "this conclusion emerged from the School of Public Health of the prestigious Harvard University." The article again juxtaposes scientific data with an overt message rejecting contemporary lifestyle and medical science.

Contemporary lifestyle is described as the source of ill health, and conventional medicine is presented as ill equipped to deal with these problems. The author offers data to support the notion that "watching violent films on TV by individuals of all age groups is detrimental to health," and claims that "there is no doubt that living in nature is the formula for longevity and good health." The reader is informed, in a polemic manner, that "the medical and scientific world is puzzled, indeed embarrassed, by its inability to discover reasons for Alzheimer's disease" and that "the incidence of those suffering from cataracts among the aged population of the western world is growing from day to day. Surgical intervention is the 'western answer' to these cases." In an item concerning the advantages of the curcumin plant, the author writes:

> yet another step in the 'return to nature' in the field of cancer as well. Cumin, the yellow component of the famous Indian spice, curry, has been 'blamed' for helping to prevent cancer of the colon. It all started with observation of people who include curry in their diet. Among these people the incidence of bowel cancer was significantly lower than among populations who do not use curry as a spice. From this point, as is common among the scientific community, the search for 'scientific proof' began. Experiments were performed on rats and findings confirmed that the cumin plant has preventive qualities. As we know—in nature we shall find our cure and not in capsules.

Unlike ideologies that employ scientific data in the service of alternative worldviews (such as creationism in the United States), the update in point represents an act of domestication in which the hegemonic institutions of conventional medicine are called on to underwrite the claims of NCM. Another interesting aspect of the update can be found in the incorporation of quotes from Maimonides. In this manner a uniquely local flavor is added to the hybrid that constitutes the contemporary construction of NCM.

The theme of Judaism and NCM is elaborated on in an article titled "Something on Chinese medicine and Judaism," written by a senior staff member described as "Master in Chinese medicine." The author establishes a connection between healing and the healer's status in the community in ancient times, mentioning the role filled by the high priest, as well as the prophets Elijah and Elisha, who resurrected the dead. The bible is mentioned as a source that contains clear instructions for the diagnosis and cure of disease, as well as explanations for the cause of disease based on morality or, rather, immorality. Similarities are pointed out between the Hassidic view of the universe and the ancient Chinese concept of the 'great world' and the 'small world.' Once again, different cultures, historical periods, and philosophies are combined to create a local hybrid. The fusion of Chinese and Hassidic concepts constitutes an apt illustration of the process of domestication.

Even though the colleges' curricula indicate the importance placed on conventional medicine and science, symbols of "otherness" are cultivated in the same framework. This is evident in the rejection of aspects of modernity apparent, for example, in the article on fashion, but also in the sense that China is perceived of as a kind of philosophical home. An educational trip to China is arranged by most colleges for advanced students and apprenticeship at a Chinese clinic provides the highlight of these excursions. Two former students who are now part of the college staff wrote an article that appeared in a college bulletin titled "China—impressions from an excursion." This article portrayed China as monumental ("the great wall of China can be seen from outer space"), and difficult to grasp: "We thought we were prepared for the fascinating journey, but when we arrived in China we started to understand that one can never be prepared enough." A photograph accompanying the article shows a Chinese doctor treating a Chinese patient with acupuncture. The caption reads: "What is more Chinese than this? Chinese acupuncture to a Chinese patient in China!" The article proceeds to describe the students' clinical experiences in China: "for two weeks we had the interesting, fascinating experience of clinical work with Chinese patients—Yes! really Chinese—who were treated by us the Israelis—according to principles of Chinese medicine." One can also read that "the progress of disposable needles has not yet reached China and we used the same needles after they had been sterilized."

The fascination and marvel at being part of a Chinese experience seem to represent a quest for authenticity—seeking out and trying to grasp the "other." The fact that most colleges employed Chinese doctors on the staff further emphasizes the quest for an "authentic" experience. This brings to mind tourism in the postmodern world (see McCannell, 1976; Urry, 1991). Although much of this Chinese spectacle could be "staged authenticity," the students of NCM did not seem to care about such fine distinctions. Moreover, they were the ones who—consciously or unconsciously—staged it. The remark concerning disposable acupuncture needles aptly illustrates the manner in which the reproduction (Chinese medicine in the West) outdoes the original.

The introductory lectures, yearbooks, curricula, and bulletins of the college show that medical science is neither abandoned nor rejected. Laboratories, diagnosis based on biomedicine, anatomy, white coats, and the prestigious Western title of doctor are retained and reproduced. At the same time, an attempt is made to capture something beyond scientific rationality. Ancient wisdom, the Orient, nature, and the "primitive other" are yearned for and reconstructed. This is the added value of NCM. It does not reject modern medicine as a grand project of modernity but enfolds an encounter between a number of cultural traditions, ultimately creating a hybrid. The acculturation inherent in this hybrid reflects a pragmatic strategy for recognition and professionalization, as well as a mirroring of the other in terms of the self.

Chapter 7

Conclusion: Familiarizing the Exotic

This study has shown how NCM in Israel is presented, represented, taught, and consumed primarily through processes of domestication. While NCM may embody countercultural ideologies that lead to differentiation, in practice its major and most successful thrust has been through selective integration and ultimately domestication. Although part of NCM's popularity might have stemmed from its import as an exotic reaction to the mainstream tenets of modern biomedical culture, the major force in establishing its presence has been hybridization and domestication. Through the mechanisms of dissemination, institutionalization, and consumption, NCM has been incorporated, appropriated, and tamed. This finding reflects both the status and power of biomedicine as well as the growing forces of consumerism. Biomedical hegemony was clearly evident in the Israeli case, for example, in the rejection of the 1991 Eilon Committee's report that recommended licensing the practice of various NCM modalities. Biomedical hegemony was also reflected in the public statement issued by the Israeli Medical Association in 1996, which opened with the words "There is no alternative medicine—there is only an alternative to medicine." Although NCM is taught in colleges, practiced in clinics, and advertised in the media, the fact remains that only MDs are legally licensed to treat people.

An additional finding that illustrates the hegemony of science, technology, and the biomedical model is the manner in which NCM is symbolically represented. NCM is marketed as a recourse to "authentic," "natural" knowledge that preceded modern biomedicine, but without regressing to what modern-day customers may perceive as primitivism. In Foucault's terms, the recourse to NCM does not involve an epistemic break. Biomedical knowledge may be contested, but it is not wholly rejected. This is apparent in various key symbols of NCM, such as the manner in which Hippocrates is brought in to the argument on the "authentic" interpretation of medicine; the combination of conventional diagnostic methods and alternative treatments; and the recourse to scientific methods to prove the effectiveness of NCM practice and/or ideology. Conversely, the absence of treatment by means of crystals or energetic healing from "mainstream" NCM probably stems from the fact that these methods are truly ex-epistemic and have not, as yet, been rephrased in current scientific terms of reference. Crystals and healing stones are therefore widely available at health food and New Age stores, as they reflect a fascination with the esoteric, but are not incorporated into institutionalized healing practices.[1]

The limiting factors acting on differentiation probably stem from the fact that "our" selves and "our" society are unavoidably entangled within the modern, taken-for-granted framework of science, technology, and progress. We can turn back to the past only from the point of view of the present. We can yearn for the old, but only in terms of the new. Ultimately, there is no going back. The "symbolic other" contained in the concept of Oriental medicine is elusive and multifaceted. Its very flexibility constitutes its potency. Manipulation of the symbols of the "other" occurs in a number of forums—the institutions of learning, the media, and the clinics.

The various forms of fusion that take place in these three settings emphasize the cultural innovation inherent in domestication. This innovation bears the marks of hegemony as well as consumption. It is innovation within the boundaries of the familiar. The domestication of NCM is comfortably tailored to the needs of the postmodern consumer. It represents "staged authenticity." NCM represents the healing of the past in the same manner that a safari represents Africa or Main Street, USA (in Disneyland) typifies a U.S. midwestern town at the end of the nineteenth century. At least some NCM consumers are comparable to postmodern tourists who take part in a quest for "staged authenticity" (McCannell, 1976). Those who (rightfully) emphasize the pain and discomfort of patients would regard the comparison to tourism as far-fetched. Nevertheless, my point is that staged authenticity is one of the motifs of the domestication of NCM in the colleges, clinics, and the media.

Domestication: Clinic, College, Media, and Patients

The clinic constitutes a physical location situated on the grounds of a large general hospital—the archetype of modern bureaucracy, science, technology, and impersonality—that sheds its conventional form to assume the categories of the alternative, a transformation achieved daily by means of sticky-tape and plastic name signs. The endocrinology clinic is transformed into a room in which reflexology is performed; the cardiology unit makes way for acupuncture needles, with the electrocardiogram machinery still occupying a dominant place in the background. The location ("part of a hospital"), the carpeting, the credit cards, the time-slots based on cost efficiency, the medical titles and the sterile, disposable needles all extend a comforting sense of familiarity and respectability often commented on by patients who had been undecided whether to seek out NCM treatment in the first place.

The staff meetings conducted at the clinic illustrated yet another fusion—that of conventional diagnostic practices with alternative treatments. This has been shown in the case studies, in which discussions were always conducted within the framework of a disease category and a diagnostic process that were part of biomedical knowledge. In these discussions the balance between the conventional/alternative parts of the fusion was sometimes disturbed, resulting in what at times appeared to be crossing the border entirely into the realm of the conventional. This was evident, for example, in the case concerning "the patient who refuses to get well." In this framework a discussion was conducted on whether it was worthwhile to refer the somatizing, hysterical patient to conventional diagnostic testing in order to prove that "nothing was wrong" and then commence alternative therapy. Even entertaining such a notion seems to negate the very philosophical basis of alternative medicine, which ideologically ascribes to the subjective and the idiosyncratic. The objective, rationalistic approach of conventional medical practice in the diagnosis of disease was employed to increase the legitimacy of NCM. Subscribing to the terms of biomedicine is imperative when opting for professionalization that is supervised by the medical establishment. In the process, the essence of **alternative** medicine is compromised while the dominance of biomedicine is reinstated. This process has also been remarked on by Margaret Lock (1990) in her study of the revival of traditional Japanese medicine in Japan. She points out that the subordination of this ancient method to modern dictates of professional referral and HMO coverage robs it of its original content.

The practice of subscribing to the terms of biomedicine creates many dilemmas for NCM. For example, many of the complaints that bothered NCM users could not be diagnosed by biomedicine. Indeed, it was often this lack of diagnosis that brought many patients to NCM in the first place. The dependence on biomedicine therefore impoverishes NCM. Within differentiation, such dependence would be unthinkable. Within domestication, however, NCM practitioners devise pragmatic strategies such as superimposing new diagnostic categories and redefining existing ones. This is observable in the manner in which common symptoms (such as coughs or rashes) are redefined as profound or superficial, or when a new etiology is suggested for these symptoms such as systemic imbalance or impaired energy flow.

Patient empowerment and partnership is an important feature in the public image of NCM, and is often mentioned in contrast to the traditional paternalistic doctor–patient relationship in biomedicine (Lupton,1997). In a study conducted on a holistic family practice clinic in the United States, Lowenburg and Davis (1994) noted less formality between health practitioners and patients and greater access to information for patients. In this clinic licensed physicians, nurses, psychologists, and nutritionists attempted to combine what they saw as the best of allopathic and holistic approaches. In contrast, my findings regarding formality do not point in one direction. Almost all doctors who worked at the NCM clinic insisted on being called "Dr." and patients did not necessarily have more access to information. I found, on the one hand, that some patients felt there was not enough authoritative guidance, whereas on the other hand, others were dissatisfied with what they perceived as too much guidance.

It transpires that NCM's general claim to "patient empowerment" should be looked at with caution and generalizations avoided. The alternative treatment itself, it should be noted, can embody both paternalism and egalitarianism. The homeopathic encounter, for example, is highly cooperative during preliminary case-taking, since the homeopath depends on the information provided by the patient. In homeopathic theory there is only one effective remedy that the practitioner prescribes, and therefore this stage of the consultation is very paternalistic and patients do not usually even learn the name of the remedy they are taking (Frank, 2002). It is likely that different NCM modalities, as well as different NCM clinics and NCM practitioners, have a different relationship with patients.

Beyond the issue of patient empowerment, studies of NCM treatment conducted in organized, institutionalized settings do seem to have some common factors. For example, Lowenberg and Davis (1994) suggest that NCM practice extends the pathogenic sphere, therefore leading to greater medicalization; and Schneirov and Gezcik (2002) have suggested that while complementary clinics located in hospitals can potentially encourage discourse between the two disciplines, there is a danger that the alternative system will be absorbed by the dominant health care system (i.e., that of conventional medicine). Notwithstanding the very different legal situation and cultural context in which these studies were conducted, these findings support my observations in the Israeli context

The College

In the institute of learning, domestication presents itself in the decor, ideology, and the curriculum. For example, a human skeleton stood in the corner of a room in which diagnosis was being demonstrated by means of the Chinese method of observing the tongue. There was no actual need for the skeleton, yet its presence signified the legacy of biomedicine. The presence of biomedicine was also felt in the curriculum (which placed emphasis on conventional medicine and science), the so-called laboratories for the demonstration of ancient techniques, and the use of scientific protocol and statistical design to prove the effectiveness of alternative or natural methods. All these point to a fusion that does not reject conventional science, but embraces it. This has also been observed by Baer et al (1998: 535). In an examination of the curricula of two American institutions in which Chinese medicine was taught, they point to "heavy emphasis on western scientific courses . . . apparently an accommodation that is required if their graduates are to pass the licensing examination for acupuncture."

Baer et al. did not, however, observe or discuss the cultural aspects of hybridization that were noted in the Israeli college. The fusion created between conventional science and NCM was not the only symbolic fusion constructed within the college studied. Another fusion, which was negotiated, was between the Oriental "other" and the

Western "self." The Oriental "other" is presented as something that the college can "authentically" represent. This authenticity is often not left to representation, but actual presentation is opted for—for example, in the form of "our man from China," the Chinese practitioner employed as an instructor at the college. The incorporation of the East is further represented through academic agreements reached with Chinese universities in addition to academic agreements with American-based colleges that grant diplomas to practice Chinese skills. However, both types of affiliation are not sufficient for accreditation in the Israeli context.

The highlight of the study program at the NCM college was the trip to China, in which the entity of "us" and the entity of the "other" would meet. This encounter, more than anything else, represents the "other" as different from the modern. At first, modernity and the ancient world seem to be on somewhat equal grounds—for example, when the Great Wall of China is described as visible from outer space. A monument of modernity, the conquest of space, and a monument of the ancient world, a man-made fortification against penetration from outside, thus become metaphorically connected. In reality, however, this encounter implies elements such as hierarchy, comparison, and even imperialism. A symbol of progress—disposable acupuncture needles—is described, for example, as "not yet having reached China." This implies the uncontested, taken-for-granted Western doctrine of biomedical progress. The "other" will eventually become "us" and "ours." In this manner the "other" is in fact tamed, rendered manageable and controllable.

The alternative trope constructed in the college also encompasses the image of "back to nature." The 'East' is connected to "the natural" by means of their supposedly shared authenticity and spirituality. The alternative trope surrounding NCM is therefore itself a hybrid construct, a "bricolage" in Claude Levi-Strauss's terms. This trope comprises elements such as "authentic" representations of the Orient, nostalgia for the potency of nature, the synchrony between man and environment, and homage to ancient and/or primitive wisdom. These elements, which are sought after and revered in the "other," are in fact a mirror image of modern society and its discontents.

The Media

NCM, as portrayed in the media, is an exaggerated image of its essential elements, both positive and negative. While the hazardous and uncertain side of NCM is depicted in "horror stories," its miraculous power of healing is conveyed through stories of "magic moments and wonder cures achieved by NCM." In both capacities, the press serves as a site for the preliminary presentation of fission, rather than fusion, between biomedical culture and NCM. While the horror stories imply the rejection of NCM, the magic moments celebrate the alternative and the uniqueness inherent in it. Obviously not all articles follow exactly the same format. All do, however, relate to conventional forms of treatment in contrast to what the alternative has to offer. In this capacity I have illustrated the representation of the "other" form of treatment as authentic, deep, and holistic when juxtaposed with conventional medicine, which is described as achieving a superficial, symptomatic cure that does not tackle the root of the problem. NCM is described as possessing the power to transcend corporeality and see what is invisible to the eye and instruments of biomedicine. Symptoms can be authentically interpreted and treated only by considering concepts such as energy and imbalance. Another symbolic construction negotiated in the media is that of purity as opposed to toxicity or pollution, regarded as elements of the modern environment. Alternative medicine offers detoxification as a means of cure. Medicines used in conventional treatment, especially antibiotics, are portrayed as a source of toxicity and iatrogenesis. Conventional medicine is described as "inundating the body with antibiotics." In this manner NCM is presented as an antidote to the perils of modern existence.

These four elements—authenticity, profundity, holism, and purity—constitute an imaginary trope, which represents an alternative to modern existence, which is perceived, in turn, as contrived, superficial, overspecialized, and toxic. A key symbol that encompasses the elements of the alternative is "nature," which is portrayed in the media as powerful, cleansing, and benevolent. This is, of course, a biased representation of "nature," one that stems directly from the nostalgic yearning for an imagined past. However, once the differences between the alternative and the scientific have been spelled out, an interesting fusion occurs. Spokespersons for alternative medicine claim that their medicine is ideally complementary to conventional medicine and proceed to make two very important claims. First, they claim that alternative medicine is in fact the true interpretation of Hippocratic law, thereby creating a historic bond between alternative and conventional medicine. Second, confidence in scientific validity is expressed; validity that might be problematic for NCM in the present, but will surely be feasible in the future, with the advance of science. One day, according to this claim, science will be advanced enough to explain the mechanisms of alternative medicine. A cultural space is therefore created, through these media stories, for the inclusion of NCM within a broader continuum of medical methods.

The media also provides an arena for the interprofessional debate between proponents of CM and NCM. In the same manner that NCM practitioners represent CM as potentially harmful, CM practitioners warn against side effects of nonconventional remedies when administered without suitable biomedical supervision. In the long run, in the interprofessional discourse conducted in the press, there is not much argument about the authority of biomedicine. It is accepted and drawn on by NCM practitioners especially those who are also MDs. Rather, the debate seems to focus on the aspiration of NCM for integration and incorporation, and the attempt of biomedicine to control this incorporation and retain its hegemony. The possibility of equivalent pluralism is not one that biomedicine views with equanimity.

The Patients

A number of theoretical explanations have been suggested to explain the growing popularity of NCM. One approach, which I called "second resort" or "limited dissatisfaction," emerged following the accumulation of data indicating that the demographic profile of NCM consumers was not unique. Hence, it was incorrect to characterize these consumers as individuals who were not fully modernized or acculturated into the mainstream of modern society. In the framework of this study, no significant demographic differences in the level of education, occupation, and income were found between patients attending the conventional clinics and those attending the NCM clinic, which is, in general, in line with the "second resort" approach.

Another explanation, which was raised in this study, suggested that recourse to NCM could be seen as part of general dissatisfaction with medicine and science in general. This trend was associated with a rejection of many of the tenets of science and technology, involvement in ecology-friendly practices, consumption of health-store products, and preoccupation with the body. One of the proponents of this approach, Mary Douglas (1994), even ventured to suggest that consumers of NCM could be characterized by a coherent, "New Age," countercultural profile. This approach, although popular, had not yet been empirically tested at the time that I performed my study on consumers and nonconsumers of NCM. Analysis of the items in the questionnaire, which examined aspects such as fascination with the cultural "other," spirituality, health consumption practices, and body maintenance, did not, on the whole, form a consistent picture. The statistical data did not provide support for the contention that using NCM is part of a general predisposition toward New Age trends.

My findings show that consumers as well as nonconsumers of NCM acknowledged the hegemony of biomedicine and were also satisfied with the representative of biomedicine with whom they were most often in contact—their primary care physician. Dissatisfaction, when expressed, was limited to the outcome of treatment for a specific problem. Moreover, patients attending the NCM clinic stressed that it was important to be treated by an MD in the framework of NCM treatment. These findings also show that many patients have resorted to a pattern of dual usage, concomitantly using both NCM and conventional medicine, or moving back and forth between the two methods. This seems to indicate that, in practice, the majority of patients do not subscribe ideologically to either one method or the other.

The sociodemographic profile of NCM users in Israel, for example, was on the whole similar to that reported in other countries (Astin, 1998; Kelner and Wellman, 1997). Indeed, the statistics showed that NCM use (indeed, dual system use) characterized patients from all walks of life. This finding replicated surveys conducted in Australia (McGregor and Peay, 1996), Canada (Kelner and Wellman, 1997; Sirois and Gick, 2002) and the United States (Druss and Rosenheck, 1999) suggesting that patients choose specific kinds of practitioners for particular problems, sometimes using a number of methods concurrently. These "smart consumers" would consult with a naturopath for colds, a chiropracter for back pain, and a conventional practitioner for an acute infection. The taken-for-granted manner in which NCM is perceived is an indicator of the success of the forces of domestication. Consulting NCM is not necessarily perceived as an esoteric choice, nor does it usually reflect a rejection of biomedicine. It is more in the line of a practical choice made among the many options that the postmodern environment offers.

Local Findings—Global Implications?

Although the ethnography presented here was conducted in Israel, the research design, the nature of the findings, and a comparison with the literature all suggest that the story told here might have global implications. Indeed, recent studies conducted in the United States, the United Kingdom, and New Zealand (Baer, 1998, 2001; Barnes, 1998; Cant and Sharma, 1999; Dew, 2000; Lowenberg and Davis, 1994; McGuire, 1988; Schneirov and Gezcik, 2002) have shown that domestication, despite the variability in medico-legal arrangements in these countries, is the dominant feature in NCM delivery. While the Israeli case should be read against the backdrop of its particular cultural context (e.g., the homogeneous perception of NCM modalities, the doctor's order, and the lack of regulation of practice and training), biomedical culture and "making sense of medicine" in local terms emerge as predominant features in the accommodation of NCM in many industrialized countries.

The domestication of NCM is not a unique phenomenon in a medical or even Western sense. Rather, it is a common strategy of the dominant culture (in our case, biomedicine) following contact with a potential challenge. Lock (1990) argued that medicine of all kinds, once incorporated within the institutionalized framework of the dominant medical system in any society, tends to act as a frame for the preservation of social order. She discusses the rationalization process that traditional herbal medicine underwent in Japan in its incorporation by biomedical practitioners. This 'rationalization' is, in fact, domestication. Similar processes of domestication are also apparent in other cultural contexts. Discussing the incorporation of Western medicine into traditional Chinese medicine, Jingfeng (1988) describes a mirror image of domestication of NCM in the West. Practitioners of Chinese medicine were aware of the impossibility of ignoring modern science, while at the same time were concerned about preserving the basic tenets of their traditional medicine. They wanted to use Western bioscience as a vehicle to advance and preserve Chinese medicine. In such interactions, the cultural "other" is constructed in local terms in order to be appropriated into the dominant, hegemonic framework. Similar processes have been observed in the adaptation of biomedicine to the meaning system of indigenous medicine in low development countries. This has been described in studies conducted by Cocks and Dold (2000) and Bledsoe and Goubaud (1985) on the manner in which Western pharmaceuticals are consumed according to the logic of local beliefs on health and treatment. In this manner the rephrasing of the "other" within the terms of the dominant culture is a means of creating order, rendering the other classifiable and understandable, thereby keeping chaos at bay (see Bauman, 1991: 9).

Why Domestication? The Interplay between Biomedical Hegemony and Consumerist Demand

Why did domestication, rather than the three other options implied by the model of acculturation and assimilation, become the dominant strategy in the case of NCM? The answer involves two major factors: the status of biomedicine and the rising popularity of NCM. Biomedicine has reached its present-day hegemony by eliminating other health systems. For example, in the thirteenth century, the Church vied for the monopoly on healing with the secular representatives of medical knowledge entrenched in the universities of Salerno or Bologna. For an extensive period during the eighteenth century in Europe, homeopathy competed with allopathy as a therapeutic system. The work of Lister and Pasteur, and the growing dependence on the scientific method, widened the gap between Western biomedicine and modalities that did not belong to this paradigm (Lupton, 1994; Turner, 1995). However, disenchantment with biomedicine reemerged in recent decades for two seemingly opposite reasons.

Along with the development of sophisticated procedures of intervention and diagnosis came iatrogenic side effects (Gabe et al., 1994; Lupton, 1995) and biomedicine was not entirely able to live up to the expectations it had created. Along with acute, heroic interventions, chronic, incurable, and terminal diseases persisted. The actual success of scientific medicine also contained the seeds of its demise. The technological progress of biomedicine introduced many costly procedures that could not be performed in accordance with consumer demand because of budgetary limitations. People were living longer due to medical interventions but were also developing chronic diseases that could not be cured. The call for cost-contained medicine was soon heard from economic institutions of the State. Cost-containment did much to erode medicine's image in the public eye, and the intervention of administrative or business considerations in clinical decisions was perceived as a threat to professional autonomy as well as to the fiduciary relationship between patient and physician (Hunter, 1991). An additional factor in the growing discontent with biomedicine was the increasing recourse to technology and sophisticated diagnostic methods, which caused alienation. The science of medicine had unsuccessfully replaced the art of medicine and the "bedside manner." This disenchantment created a cultural climate that was less receptive to the outright rejection of NCM solely on the grounds of the superiority of the scientific method.

In this climate, two interlinked forces came into play. From the outside, forces of globalization made alternative methods more accessible. From within, there were professional voices that called for greater flexibility and diversity, perhaps as part of the postmodern collapse of boundaries. As a result, biomedicine underwent two processes: fragmentation and accommodation. In a manner similar to the domestication of religion illustrated by Sered (1988), biomedicine became fragmented from within. As different groups within medicine started to voice different opinions, biomedicine in general started to adopt a discourse that was not entirely "scientific," at least according to the positivistic criteria of the past. For example, the conceptualization of the discourse of neuropsychoimmunology and the biopsychosocial model of etiology rephrased the psychosomatic in scientific terms. Well-known doctors such as Deepak Chopra (1999) or scientists such as Candace Pert (1999) pushed the borders of the materialist, Cartesian view of medicine into the domain of mind-body interactions that could not quite be explained, but could perhaps be controlled. Especially interesting in this capacity is the potential for the individual to take responsibility or even to "be blamed" for the state of his or her health. This latter issue has been observed by Lowenberg and Davis (1994) in their discussion of the manner in which NCM extends the scope of medicalization. The conceptual similarity between this approach and the holistic model perpetrated by alternative medicine is remarkable, and strengthens the sense of a common cultural context, in which both conventional and alternative medicine are now developing and perhaps will converge in the future.

Further illustration of the fragmenting processes occurring within bio-medicine can be observed in a study conducted by Schachter et al (1993) that showed that Israeli general practitioners were willing to refer patients to alternative practitioners even though they did not believe that alternative medicine had a scientific basis. The referral of patients to NCM modalities by general practitioners has been observed in a number of other countries (Knipschild et al.,1990; White et al., 1997). Moreover, the fact that many MDs practice NCM modalities and

Conclusion

publically promote its philosophy and ideology further indicates that biomedicine is indeed changing from within. This is also observable on the structural level—for example, by the fact that NCM is taught in a number of medical schools. Therefore, while it appears that NCM is adjusting to the dominant medical paradigm, it would be simplistic to view this process as unidirectional. The host culture is also affected, although to a lesser degree. However, one can witness a shift in the hegemonic as well as the challenging paradigm. It is interesting to note that whereas the proponents of NCM within biomedicine can be seen as liberal forces that contribute to the legitimacy of NCM in the public eye, they are actually quite instrumental in extending medicalization as more and more spheres come under the scrutiny of the medical gaze.

It is interesting to recall, in this context, the Israeli Medical Association's statement that "there is no alternative medicine—only an alternative to medicine." This statement opened the manifesto issued by the association in 1997, in response to the recommendation to license NCM practitioners. I have previously read this statement as a blatant indication of the exclusive hegemony of biomedicine. However, another reading can be offered at this point. "There is no alternative medicine, only an alternative to medicine" could also mean that "alternative medicine" is but a label, since all medicine is about healing and curing. Seen in this broadest sense, there is indeed only "one medicine"—that which seeks to cure and heal. While this reading was not intended by the association, it could still characterize certain physicians who are pragmatic in their quest to provide an answer to a patient's complaint. Moreover, the co-optation of the alternative, at least in part, into biomedical practice tames and domesticates it as complementary, instead of having to deal with it as a full-fledged adversary.

No doubt it was the phenomenon of consumerist demand in Israel—with which nobody could argue—that pushed NCM out of the categories of low assimilation (rejection, selective integration). Fueled by consumerist demand, NCM could flourish in two categories: differentiation and domestication. The option of differentiation (i.e., developing an alternative ideology) did not fail because of biomedical resistance alone but most probably because the familiarization of NCM modalities by cultural brokers provided a "safe" option for experiencing the foreign entities of NCM. In this manner, the pluralistic recourse to a variety of therapeutic modalities was facilitated by the fact that the cultural price was not too high. The domesticating processes that rendered the foreign familiar can thus be seen as the basic drive behind patients' so-called rational, taken-for-granted, health choices that maximize the best of both worlds (CM and NCM), and provide a cultural explanation for this type of health maintenance behavior. The explanation of "smart consumerism" therefore rests on processes of domestication that slowly brought about a shift in the hegemonic paradigm that, in turn, legitimated NCM and fueled consumer demand. A self-propagating circle then emerged in which public demand resulted in the establishment of complementary clinics, in which MDs were involved, which, in turn, amplified public demand.

The "Other" Appropriated and the "Other" Rejected

Bauman (1992a) speaks about "the astonishing ability of the postmodern habitat to absorb dissent and avant-garde criticism, and deploy them as sources of its own renewed strength" (p. 185). This study both validates and extends Bauman's contention. I have shown how NCM (a form of potential dissent) has been absorbed and domesticated by biomedicine. This validates Bauman's claim about the flexibility of the postmodern habitat. However, in contrast to Bauman's view of the "end of ideology" in the postmodern, this study shows that for all its flux, the postmodern—if it indeed exists—contains islands of hegemony. Biomedicine is still very much a metanarrative within the Israeli milieu. In Israel, the exclusivity of biomedicine is maintained by strict laws such as the doctors' order. And even though this order is not strictly enforced, the development of NCM in Israel has been along biomedical lines—not because of formal enforcement but probably due to the informal realization of limits decided on by cultural brokers. If we adopt the postmodern approach of fragmentation, we encounter a paradox: How can the metanarrative of biomedicine still exist within a fragmented postmodern environment, which nurtures a multitude of competing, equivalent narratives, where "everything goes"?

The postmodern world has been described as a development, or outcome, of the modern world, although not all writers have felt comfortable with the term "postmodern" since it implies the end of modernity (Harvey, 1991; Jameson, 1991). For this reason, Giddens (1991), for example, has preferred the terms "high" versus "late" modernity. Postmodernity as a period, according to Bauman's (1991) conceptualization, is characterized by self-reflexivity, which has replaced the modern thrust for unitary order, accountability, and rationality.

In another book, Bauman (1992a) distinguishes between two types of "identity seekers": The postmodernist nomads and the Protestant (modernist) "pilgrims through life." This distinction between nomads and pilgrims is relevant to the "dual use" strategy that characterizes today's NCM consumers. It would have been rational to expect single use or "loyalty" from the modernist "pilgrims." However, postmodern "nomads" are not committed to any single path, as the very essence of "nomadism" dictates dual use or even multiple uses. In other words, even if biomedicine still represents a modernist hegemony, the postmodern consumer is already a "nomad." The metaphor of the nomad brings to mind another metaphor that I have alluded to before, that of the tourist. As nomads or tourists, smart consumers of NCM wander through hospitals and clinics. Lacking a distinctive cultural profile or ideology, many NCM consumers are using consumption itself as a source of identity or a "lifestyle." Such identity, however, is not ideologically fixed (hence refuting the 'differentiation' category) but opportunistic and often fickle. In Giddens's words (1991: 14), "Late modernity is a post-traditional order, in which the question, 'How shall I live?' has to be answered in day-to-day decisions about how to behave, what to wear and what to eat—and many other things—as well as interpreted within the temporal unfolding of self-identity."

NCM and the Postmodern Body

In the beginning of this book I suggested a linkage between the rising popularity of NCM and the "return of the body" in postmodern consumer culture. The body has become a primary locus for individual control and self-realization (Hannerz, 1996; Turner, 1996; Shilling, 1993) in an increasingly hostile and unstable postmodern environment. NCM, which is perceived as a more caring and intimate alternative to the alienated anonymity of biomedicine, reflects for many a nostalgic return to a romanticized past when people relied on nature and community rather than on science, medicine, and technology (Coward, 1993). This new concern with the body is in my view part of the domestication of NCM, since it highlights how NCM is appropriated by a very local discourse of the body.

The postmodern concern with the body has opened up a symbolic space in which people can also express dissatisfaction with contemporary society and feel they are personally "doing something about it" by grooming, tending, feeding, and molding their bodies in a certain way. NCM therefore claims to be a source of empowerment, restoring a sense of personal control over the body (and soul) as well as providing a sense of belonging to an "ideological community." Evidently, the "ideological community" constructed around NCM, depicted in such a manner, was in many cases an imagined community that hinged on sporadic transactions. However, such imagined communities are not unique to NCM. They have already become an integral part of global consumerism, as in thematic tourism, food fairs, media events, world expositions, sports events, and music performances.

Part of the popularity of NCM is derived from the failure of biomedicine to treat and cure chronic diseases and psychosomatic problems. Patients suffering from chronic or psychosomatic conditions seek out NCM because it can offer them something that biomedicine does not: an explanation and a remedy. Whereas biomedicine rested on a bureaucratic and impersonal outlook in which the body is objectified and fragmented into bits and pieces according to the medical specialty of the attending physician, NCM disseminated itself as an alternative discourse, in which the body as a whole receives personal attention and the human subject regains a central and active place in the therapeutic interaction.

Attitudes toward the body are presumably an important aspect of the popularity of NCM. A host of studies have analyzed postmodern Western society as governed by consumerist fashions and spectacles in which the body plays an important role (Chaney, 1993; Ewen and Ewen, 1982; Glassner, 1989). Could it be that NCM has become one such fashion as part of the postmodern spectacle of the body? NCM could be seen in this context as a consumerist means for regaining personal control against the biomedical government of the body. The popularity of NCM methods that do not treat diseases but rather concentrate on health maintenance by helping one to "feel good" and "stay in shape" could be viewed as part of a fast-growing business that includes health clubs and spas, cosmetic surgery, organic and diet foods, and various exercising fads. Discussing fitness and the postmodern self, Glassner (1989: 183) wrote that "Even when fitness is pursued privately, in one's home, the body is commonly experienced by way of conceptual looking glasses—by how it is interpreted in comparison to images of bodies in the media, and how it is commented upon by others."

The body serves as a key symbol and an organizing context of meaning for the practitioners and users of NCM. I have argued that, on the whole, NCM does indeed offer a perspective on the body that differs from that of conventional medicine (Fadlon, 2004b). The popularity of NCM could therefore imply resistance to the gaze or even demedicalization. Bryan Turner (1992) claimed that in our "somatic society" major political and personal issues are both problematized in the body and expressed through it and Emily Martin (1994) has shown how images of the body in America reflect a profound shift from the early twentieth-century paradigm of a collectivist "Fordist body" that centered on standardized production, into a consumerist paradigm of individual "flexible specialization." If Martin is correct, then the popularity of NCM could also be part of a new paradigm that is reflected in the body.

In contrast to the fragmenting gaze of biomedicine, alternative medicine presented itself through the ideal of holism. However, the paradigmatic challenge of alternative medicine was domesticated, and its original ideology was rephrased in familiar terms. Thus the key metaphor of "energy" appeared and claimed a leading role in the Western staging of NCM. Through the emphasis on entities such as energy, chakras, or auras the "holistic body" (an entity already fragmented by the medical gaze) dematerialized in order to attain new coherence. However, a closer look shows that this "alternative" view of the body based on the dual tenets of holism and dematerialization is not as ex-paradigmatic as we might have thought. It is part of the dominant biomedical paradigm in which the boundaries of the body are already becoming increasingly fragmented and blurred (Turner, 1996). This is observable, for example, in postmodern medical technologies such as in-vitro fertilization, video consultation, genetic engineering, and transplantation, all of which are techniques that redraw the boundaries of the physical body.

According to Williams (1997), advances in medical science and technology have made our bodies increasingly plastic; they can be molded, synthesized, and engineered. Technologies of cosmetic surgery greatly expand the limits of how the body may be restyled and reshaped (Davis, 1994). The body also becomes increasingly bionic (or synthesized) with cardiac pacemakers, plastic valves, titanium hips, polymer blood vessels, electronic eye and ear implants, and even polyurethane hearts (Balsamo, 1995; Haraway, 1991; Synott, 1993). The body also becomes increasingly engineered through new forms of genetics. One of the latest developments is virtual medicine where, instead of the patient's body being at the center, we find instead "multiple images and codings" whereby the body is endlessly "simulated" (Frank, 1992: 83). According to Williams's (1997: 1047) description of the change in the biomedical outlook, "a modernist concern with corporeality is slowly but surely giving way to a postmodernist concern with hyper-reality."

The "energy" (whether metaphor or reality) characterizing the NCM narrative is no longer a stranger within the postmodern context of hyperreality. It can be added to the now-familiar list of postmodern biomedical concepts that deal with virtual bodies. One major objection to this hypothesis, however, is that NCM's "energy," unlike biomedical concepts, cannot be measured by objective means. In the meantime (until biomedicine finds a measure for the vital energy of NCM), practices for diagnosing, balancing, and enhancing energy levels can subject the individual to even greater scrutiny and control. The focus on "energy" provides a new locus of surveillance as NCM therapists seek out impaired energy flow or refer to stimulation of vital forces. This points to a paradox inherent in the original promise of NCM. Instead of freeing patients from medical control by empowering them to understand and take care of their bodies (demedicalization), an extended process of control is at work here in the form of more extensive medicalization of the body. NCM has conceptualized additional fields through which the body, as well as the patient, can be surveyed and controlled by a new class of experts.

We are in the midst of a process. The popularity of NCM is still on the rise as it continues to entrench itself as a taken-for-granted option in the health care market. One possibility is that it could continue to develop in the path of domestication and become ever more 'complementary' to conventional medicine. In the process, it could also constitute a Trojan horse that would change biomedicine from within. As more MDs become exposed to NCM and its growing popularity among health consumers, and NCM is taught at medical schools, biomedicine could undergo a paradigmatic shift that would promote the inclusion of NCM into biomedical practice, possibly even hospital wards. The discourse of 'energy' and 'vital forces' would then become part of the gaze of biomedicine. Such dual transformation—the complete domestication of NCM along with a parallel change in biomedicine—would be the culmination of dedifferentiation, that all-consuming power of postmodern consumer culture. If such a flattening out of difference between NCM and biomedicine were indeed to take place, it would constitute a victory of postmodernism over one of the last strongholds of modern positivism, biomedicine. Conversely, NCM could start to develop along a different path, leading away from acculturation and pressing toward the creation of islands of counterculture. Another viable option would be a combination of these possibilities, with some branches of NCM (e.g., chiropractic and acupuncture) becoming more domesticated while others (reflexology and classic homeopathy) retain their original theoretical premises. Using the model of assimilation and acculturation, the anthropology of medicine can follow these future developments among the many actors on the stage. "Change" remains the one thing of which we can be certain.

Appendix: NCM Modalities Available at the Clinic

The NCM clinic I studied offered its patients leaflets containing information on relevant methods of treatment. Each method was written up by a therapist-practitioner from that discipline. It is interesting to note that although these printed handouts, which constituted a page-long description of each method, were supposed to be readily available to patients, they rarely ever were. Patients who requested written material (not many did) about a certain modality usually did so after the first consultation with the sorting doctor. This was normally in order to read up about the method to which they had been referred. Because clinic policy required more or less fair distribution of the patients among the various practitioners, perhaps unlimited access to information about the methods could have created demand that the clinic would not have been able to handle. In general, however, when a patient specifically requested a particular method, the sorting doctor would generally make an effort to accommodate this request. Leaflets were not available for the following modalities, although they were available at the clinic: traditional Chinese medicine, acupuncture, and shiatsu.

Chiropractic was founded by Daniel David Palmer in 1895 and derived its name from Greek, meaning "done by hand." The pamphlet states at the outset that it is a "manual medicine that does not utilize medication, and is recognized by the Ministry of Health." The chiropractor is described as a graduate of one of the twenty recognized colleges throughout the world, primarily in the United States, that offer a six-year program that includes basic studies in conventional medicine with specialization in chiropractic. In this manner a claim is made for near-medical status and all chiropractors go by the title "Dr." The fact that their profession is recognized by the Ministry of Health is an additional factor in the relatively high status enjoyed by chiropractors in the pecking order of NCM. In the handout, chiropractic is described as dealing with the "stabilization and balance of the vertebrae of the spinal column in order to enable the nervous system to function properly in all parts of the body."

Medicinal herbs are described as a mode of treatment suitable for women, men, and children, the young and the old who are suffering from problems that have not been adequately treated by conventional medicine. The description of the system creates a holistic view of processes of disease and health. "There are many disturbances and diseases in which a particular organ is affected by malfunctioning of another organ in the body which means that both organs have to be treated with the appropriate herbs. For example, when one treats migraines with medicinal herbs, one prescribes herbs for the nervous system, for the blood vessels which contract and cause the onset of a migraine and in addition to all that, also herbs for other systems in the body which cause the outbreak of migraines due to their malfunction." Beyond this holistic view of the interconnectedness of the various systems in the body, various combinations of herbs are described as having an antibiotic effect on the body and others as having an effect on the body's resistance. In the words of the pamphlet, "children who suffer from recurrent bouts of illness also receive herbs which raise the level of the body's immunity, in this way treating an infection as well as preventing future contagion."

Paula technique is described in the brochure as "teaching people to help themselves through realization of the potential inherent in their bodies. In follow-ups of patients and students over the past 50 years we have discovered again and again that the body has the potential to heal itself and maintain its state of health." The Paula technique assumes an interconnectedness of various groups of muscles in the body. Exercising one group will invariably effect other groups. The list of physical complaints that the method can help cure is a long one. The method, however, is also useful in the "maintenance of vitality and a better quality of life."

The Meyer method is based on "cleansing the body of poisons which have accumulated in the course of the years and teaching correct eating habits." Cleansing the body of toxins leads to expulsion of large amounts of waste materials that have accumulated in the body and the intestine in the course of time, and are responsible for many ailments from which we suffer.

Homeopathy is described as a "medical method based on principles and laws discovered by a doctor called Dr. Samuel Hahnemann who lived in Germany 200 years ago." Hahnemann and his successors are depicted as carrying out experiments that led to finding over 2,000 medicines that, when suited to the patient, bring about deep changes in the physical as well as the mental–spiritual state. These changes are always in the direction of balance and do not change the individual's character. "According to the Homeopathic concept, the patient's symptoms do not constitute the sickness itself, but rather an expression of a disturbance on a deeper plane. The effect of the Homeopathic remedy is on a profound, root level which renders its action to be deep and inclusive.

We may therefore witness recovery—or a genuine improvement in symptoms (in contrast to a situation of external and artificial disappearance of complaints)." The homeopathic remedy is described as "activating the body's internal powers of healing, resulting in a genuine rather than an external effect." Homeopathy is presented as a method suited to treat "almost any problem on condition that the damage already caused to the patients is reversible and reparable. The success of treatment depends on receiving all existing information on the patient and correctly choosing the exact remedy."

Reflexology is described as a therapeutic method belonging to a group of therapeutic methods based on a holistic worldview—a view of the body and soul as one unit. The body is described as functioning on the principle of polarity with the flow of energy connecting the poles. Deep massage of the soles of the feet and pressure applied at certain points lead to renewal of the energy flow, causing the body to receive a boost toward renewed balance.

Nutrition: The description of the therapeutic scope of nutrition is introduced by describing a WHO report that estimates that nutrition is a cardinal risk factor in the development of disease in the modern world. The contribution of nutrition to disease processes is not limited only to consumption of calories and fat on the one hand, or nutrient deficiency on the other, but to the realization that fortifying the diet with certain nutrient factors such as vitamins, minerals, and food additives contributes to the prevention of, or minimization of, damage from factors causing illnesses in the Western world. Nutrition, however, is not only described as contributing to physical illness, but its therapeutic claim is extended to include mental well-being as well. Under the heading "The Nutritional Approach to Behavioral Problems" nutrition is described as having an effect on one's mental state, performance, and coping with the environment. The body can be fortified and stress decreased. Self-control and efficient behavior can be attained. This is also the basis for the nutritional approach to the treatment of behavioral problems in children such as hyperactivity, dyslexia, problems in learning, communication, and adaptation. Behavioral problems in adults such as anxiety, a tendency to depression, fatigue, tension, irritability, and sleep disorders can also be treated by means of nutrition. The therapeutic direction assumed presumes that instead of repressing the sickness, the symptoms should be utilized as a guide to planning the type of nutrition that will create the chemistry in the body that will facilitate self healing.

Natural-Holistic Medicine: This discipline, represented by a single MD, utilizes the informative handout to directly address the patient. "Dear Convalescer," he writes, "the purpose of this letter is to clarify the nature of the service which you are about to receive as well as the therapeutic philosophy behind it. Today, with the extensive variety of therapeutic approaches, I feel that it is important that the health consumer will understand what lies in store for him/her in our mutual enterprise. I believe that health is first and foremost the result of a healthy way of life. Health constitutes the natural state of the body when it is supplied with the necessary prerequisites and on condition that obstacles to the maintenance of this natural state are removed. The prerequisites for good health can be found in the field of nutrition, movement, rest, clean environment and psychological-emotional balance. The body is imprinted with the wisdom and the knowledge to heal itself and it does it better than any doctor or medicine."

The practitioner ends the brochure with the following promise:

> In my cooperation with convalescers I will try and identify the reason lying at the source of the problem presented by the patient and I will try to treat it and not the symptoms, whilst attempting to alleviate suffering and pain.
>
> I perceive my work with convalescers as team work, in which I function as a guide, companion and teacher. A cardinal principle for me in our mutual relationship is the issue of delegating responsibility and transferring power to the patient.
>
> My tendency is to avoid conventional medications as much as possible. On the other hand we will concentrate on aspects of lifestyle such as nutrition, physical exercise and rest, mental health, prevention of environmental toxication. I will use, as necessary, additional methods of natural healing such as medicinal herbs, hydrotherapy, guided imagination, various meth-

ods of relaxation, work on soft tissue, manipulation of the spinal cord and Homeopathy in acute conditions.

In the event that what has been said above touches you, I will be glad to embark on cooperation.

Wishing you health and happiness, Dr. D.

Notes

Chapter 3

1. I am indebted to Henry Abramowitch for pointing out that the actual move from one physical and therapeutic locus to another has repercussions for patients and therapists alike. Abramowitch has elaborated on this point in his article "Temenos lost, or: when the clinic moves." This article set me thinking about what changed could have been made (but were not) in the clinic's decor when it moved from shared rooms to its own quarters.

Chapter 5

1. The popular media plays an important role in the dissemination of information on health, illness, and medicines. A study conducted by the internal control department of the hospital to which the clinic was adjacent showed that during the first year of activity, 59% of the patients who had been treated at the clinic stated that they had heard of the clinic through the popular media. Five years later, in a questionnaire distributed in the framework of this study, 11.3% of the respondents stated that they had heard of the clinic through the media. The relative decrease in the number of patients actually attending the clinic following media exposure does not minimize the role of the media in the dissemination of information on health and medicine. In the same questionnaire, 25.2% of the respondents reported that the media constituted a primary source of information on NCM.

Chapter 6

1. In the course of my fieldwork friends often awarded me the rather dubious title of "expert" in NCM and used to ask me for recommendations of practitioners. They also discussed with me treatments received and practitioners consulted. One friend, who was seeing a naturopath, said: "It's difficult to know if she really is an MD or not. There are so many framed documents and certificates on the wall that it's difficult to make it out. She calls herself

"Dr." but I think she might be a PhD. I don't want to ask her outright in case she gets offended." Another friend conducted a heated argument with me on the biomedical status of an acupuncturist who was treating her. I knew for sure that he was not an MD, although he did like to create the impression that he had attained this status. "But he writes 'Dr.' on his prescription pads and receipts," my friend ventured in his defense. Indeed he did, but had neglected to qualify the use of the title "Dr." by adding the letters OMD after his name. In general, both these practitioners had made the effort to convey the impression that they were in fact MDs, which emphasizes the cultural and professional importance they afford to the title.

Chapter 7

1. The theoretical knowledge on which the potency of stones is based is probably most suited to the first episteme describe by Foucault, in which legends attributed to an object fulfilled an explanatory function equivalent to the object's morphological elements.

References

Abramovitch, Henry. 1997. "Temenos lost, or: when the clinic moves," *Journal of Analytical Psychology* 42, 569–584.

Appadurai, Arjun, and Carol Breckenridge. 1988. "Why Public Culture?," *Public Culture* 1, 1:5–9.

Armstrong, D. 1987. "Bodies of knowledge: Foucault and the problem of human anatomy." In Graham Scrambler (ed.), *Sociological Theory and Medical Sociology*. London: Tavistock.

Astin, J. A. 1998. "Why patients use alternative medicine," *JAMA* 279, 19:1548–1553.

Baer, Hans. 2001. *Biomedicine and Alternative Healing Systems in America—Issues of Class, Race, Ethnicity and Gender*. Madison: University of Wisconsin Press.

Baer, Hans, Merrill Singer, and Ida Susser. 1997. *Medical Anthropology and the World System—A Critical Perspective*. Westport: Bergin and Garvey.

Baer, Hans, Cindy Jen, Lucia Tanassi, Christopher Tsia, and Helen Wahbeh. 1998. "The drive for professionalization in acupuncture: A preliminary view from the San Francisco Bay Area," *Social Science and Medicine* 46, 4–5:533–537.

Bakx, K. 1991. "The 'eclipse' of folk medicine in "western society," *Sociology of Health and Illness* 13, 1:20–38.

Balsamo, Anne. 1995. *Technologies of the Gendered Body: Cyborg Women*. Durham: Duke University Press.

Barnes, L. 1998. "The pychologizing of Chinese healing practices in the United States," *Culture, Medicine and Psychiatry* 22:413–443.

Bauman, Zygmunt. 1991. *Modernity and Ambivalence*. Cambridge: Polity Press.

———. 1992a. *Intimations of Postmodernity*. London: Routledge.

———. 1992b. *Mortality and Immortality and Other Life Strategies*. Cambridge: Polity Press.

Berg, M. 1995. "Turning a practice into a science: Reconceptualizing postwar medical practice," *Social Studies of Science* 25:437–476.

References

Berger, A. A. 1997. *Narratives in Popular Culture, Media, and Everyday Life.* London: Sage.

Bernstein, Judith H., and Judith T. Shuval. 1997. "Nonconventional medicine in Israel: Consultations patterns of the Israeli population and attitudes of primary care physicians," *Social Science and Medicine* 44, 9:1341–1348.

Berry, J. 1990. "Acculturation as varieties of adaptation." In A. M. Padilla (ed.), *Acculturation: Theory, Models and Some New Findings.* Boulder: Westview Press.

Berry, J., U. Kim, and P. Boski. 1988. "Psychological acculturation of immigrants." In Y. Kim and F. B. Gudykunst (eds.), *Cross-cultural Adaptation.* Beverly Hills: Sage, pp. 62–89.

Bibeau, Gilles. 1985. "From China to Africa: The same impossible synthesis between traditional and western medicines," *Social Science and Medicine* 21, 8:937–943.

Bilu, Yoram. 1977. "General characteristics of referrals to traditional healers in Israel," *The Israel Annals of Psychiatry and Related Disciplines* 15:245–252.

———. 1979. "Demonic explanations of disease among Moroccan Jews in Israel," *Culture, Medicine and Psychiatry* 3, 4:363–380.

———. 1980. "The Moroccan demon in Israel: The case of 'evil spirit disease,'" *Ethos* 8, 1:24–39.

Bilu, Yorum, and E. Ben-Ari. 1992. "The making of modern saints," *American Ethnologist* 4:672–688.

Bilu, Yoram, Eliezer Witztum, and Onno Van der Hart. 1990. "Paradise regained: 'Miraculous healing' in an Israeli psychiatric clinic," *Culture, Medicine and Psychiatry* 14, 1:105–127.

Bishaw, M. 1991. "Promoting traditional medicine in Ethiopia: A brief historical review of government policy," *Social Science and Medicine* 33, 2:193–200.

Bledsoe, C. H., and M. F. Goubaud. 1985. "The reinterpretation of western pharmaceuticals among the Mende of Sierra Leone," *Social Science and Medicine* 21, 3:275–282.

Bodeker, Gerard. 2001. "Lessons on integration from the developing world's experience," *British Medical Journal*, 322, 7279:164–171.

Bury, M., and J. Gabe. 1994. "Television and medicine: Medical dominance or trial by the media?" In J. Gabe, D. Kelleher, and G. Williams (eds.), *Challenging Medicine.* London: Routledge.

References

Cant S. L., and M. Calnan. 1991. "On the margins of the medical marketplace? An exploratory study of alternative practitioners' perceptions," *Sociology of Health and Illness* 13, 1:39–57.

Cant, Sarah, and Ursula Sharma. 1996. "Demarcation and transformation within homeopathic knowledge: A strategy of professionalization," *Social Science and Medicine* 42, 4:579–588.

———. 1999. *A new medical pluralism? Alternative medicine, doctors, patients and the state.* London: UCL Press, Taylor and Francis Group.

Chaney, D. 1993. *Fictions of Collective Life.* London: Routledge.

Chopra, Deepak. 1999. *Quantam Healing: Exploring the Frontiers of Mind Body Medicine.* New York: Random House.

Cockerham, W. 1986. *Medical Sociology.* Englewood Cliffs, NJ: Prentice-Hall.

Cocks, M., and A. Dold. 2000. "The role of 'African Chemists' in the health care system of the Eastern Cape province of South Africa," *Social Science and Medicine* 51:1505–1515.

Comaroff, J. 1993. "The diseased heart of Africa." In S. Lindenbaum and M. Lock (eds.), *Knowledge Power and Practice.* Berkeley: UCLA Press.

Coward, Rosalind. 1993. "The myth of alternative medicine." In A. Beattie, M. Gott, L. Jones, and M. Sidell (eds.), *Health and Wellbeing.* London: Macmillan.

Davis, K. 1994. *Reshaping the Female Body: The Dilemmas of Cosmetic Surgery.* London: Routledge.

Denzin, Norman K. 1978. *The Research Act.* New York: McGraw-Hill.

Der Derian, J., and M. J. Shapiro (eds.). 1989. *International/Intertextual Relations: Postmodern Readings of World Politics.* Lexington: D. C. Heath.

Dew, K. 2000. "Deviant insiders: Medical acupuncturists in New Zealand," *Social Science and Medicine* 50:1785–1795.

Douglas, M. 1994. "The construction of the physician: A cultural approach to medical fashions." In S. Budd and U. Sharma (eds.), *The Healing Bond.* London: Routledge.

Druss, B. G., and R. A. Rosenheck. 1999. "Association between use of unconventional therapies and conventional medical services," *JAMA* 282, 7:651–656.

Eisenberg, D. M., R. B. Davis, S. L. Ettner, et al. 1998. "Trends in alternative medicine use in the US, 1990–97: Results of a follow-up national survey," *JAMA* 280:1569–1575.

Eisenberg, D. M., R. C. Kessler, C. Foster, F. E. Norlock, D. R. Calkins, and T. L. Delbanco. 1993. "Unconventional medicine in the U.S.—Prevalence, costs and patterns of use," *New England Journal of Medicine* 328:246–252.

Eisenstadt, S. N. 1985. *The Transformations of Israeli Society: An Essay in Interpretation*. London: Weidenfeld and Nicholson.

Ewen, S., and E. Ewen. 1982. *Channels of Desire*. New York: McGraw-Hill.

Fadlon, J. 2004a. "Unrest in Utopia—Israeli patients' dissatisfaction with non-conventional medicine," *Social Science and Medicine* 58, 12:2421–2429.

———. 2004b. "Meridians, chakras and psycho-neuro-immunology: The dematerializing body and the domestication of alternative medicine," *Body and Society* 10, 4.

Fadlon, J., M. Granek, I. Roziner, M. Weingarten, and N. Lewin-Epstein. 2003. "Familiarity breeds discontent: Senior hospital doctors' attitudes towards complementary alternative medicine," unpublished manuscript. Tel Aviv: Sapir Foundation.

Farge, J. 1977. "A review of the findings from 'three generations' of Chicano health care behavior," *Social Science Quarterly* 58, 3:407–411.

Featherstone, Mike. 1991. *Consumer Culture and Postmodernism*. London: Sage.

——— (ed.). 1992. *The Body and Social Theory*. London: Sage.

———. 1995. *Undoing Culture*. London: Sage.

Finkler, K. 1981. "A comparative study of health seekers: Or why do some people go to doctors rather than to spiritualist healers?," *Medical Anthropology* 5, 4:383–424.

Fisher, P., and A. Ward. 1994. "Complementary medicine in Europe," *British Medical Journal* 309:107–110.

Foucault, Michel. 1967. *Madness and Civilization*. New York: Random House.

Frank, A. 1992. "Twin nightmares of the medical simulacrum: Baudrillard and Cronenberg." In W. Stearns and W. Chalouplea (eds.), *Jean Baudrillard: The Disappearance of Art and Politics*. London: Macmillan.

Frank, R. 2002. "Homeopath and patient—A dyad of harmony?," *Social Science and Medicine* 55:1285–1296.

Furnham, A., and J. Forey. 1994. "The attitudes, behaviors and beliefs of patients of conventional vs. complementary (alternative) medicine," *Journal of Clinical Psychology* 50, 3:458–469.

Gabe, J., D. Kelleher, and G. Williams. 1994. "Understanding medical dominance in the modern world." In J. Gabe, D. Kelleher, and G. Williams (eds.), *Challenging Medicine*. London: Routledge.

References

Gergen, K., and M. Gergen. 1988. "Narrative and the self as relationship," *Advances in Experimental Social Psychology* 21:17–55.

Giddens, Anthony. 1991. *Modernity and Self-Identity*, Stanford: Stanford University Press.

———. 1994. *Beyond Left and Right*. London: Polity Press.

Glassner, Barry. 1989. "Fitness and the post-modern self," *Journal of Health and Social Behavior* 30:180–191.

Goldstein, D. 1988. "Holistic physicians and family practitioners, differences and implications for health policy," *Social Science and Medicine* 26, 8:853–861.

Good, Byron J. 1994. *Medicine, Rationality, and Experience: An Anthropological Perspective*. Cambridge: Cambridge University Press.

Gray, D. 1985. "The treatment strategies of arthritis sufferers," *Social Science and Medicine* 21, 5:507–515.

Grinstein, O., A. Elhayany, A. Goldberg, and S. Shvarts. 2002. "Complementary medicine in Israel," *The Journal of Alternative and Complementary Medicine,* 8, 4:437–443.

Gubrium, Jaber F. 1988. *Analyzing Field Reality—Qualitative Research Methods #8* Newbury Park: Sage.

Hall, Stuart. 1992. "Encoding, Decoding." In Simon During (ed.), *The Cultural Studies Reader*. London: Blackwell.

Hannerz, Ulf. 1989. "Notes on the Global Ecumene," *Public Culture* 1, 2:66–75.

———. 1992. *Cultural Complexity*. New York: Columbia University Press.

———. 1996. *Transnational Connections*. London: Routledge.

Haram, L. 1991. "Tswana medicine in interaction with bio-medicine," *Social Science and Medicine* 33, 2:167–175.

Haraway, Donna. 1991. *Simians, Cyborgs and Women*. London: Free Association Books.

Hare, Martha L. 1993. "The emergence of an Urban US Chinese medicine," *Medical Anthropology Quarterly* 7:30–49.

Harvey, David. 1989. *The Condition of Postmodernity: An Enquiry into the Origins of Cultural Change*. Oxford: Basil Blackwell.

Hilgartner, Stephen. 1990. "The dominant view of popularization: Conceptual problems, political uses," *Social Studies of Science* 20:519–539.

Hood, Jacqueline, and Koberg, Christine. 1994. "Patterns of differential assimilation and acculturation for women in business organizations," *Human Relations* 47, 2:159–171.

Huizer, Gerritt. 1987. "Indigenous healers and western dominance: Challenge for social scientists?," *Social Compass* 34, 4:415–436.

Hunter, D. 1991. "Managing medicine: A response to the 'crisis,'" *Social Science and Medicine* 32, 4:441–449.

Jameson, Frederic. 1991. *Postmodernism, or, the Cultural Logic of Late Capitalism*. Durham: Duke University Press.

Jingfeng, C. 1988. "Integration of traditional Chinese medicine with western medicine—Right or wrong?," *Social Science and Medicine* 27, 5:521–529.

Katriel, Tamar. 1986. *Talking Straight: Dugri Speech in Israeli Sabra Culture*. Cambridge: Cambridge University Press.

———. 1991. *Communal Webs: Culture and Communication in Israel*. Albany: State University of New York Press.

Katz, Elihu, and Michael Gurevitch. 1976. *The Secularization of Leisure: Culture and Communication in Israel*. London: Faber and Faber.

Kelner, Merrijoy, and Beverly Wellman. 1997. "Health care and consumer choice: Medical and alternative therapies," *Social Science and Medicine* 45, 2:203–212.

King, Anthony D. (ed.). 1991. *Culture, Globalization and the World-System*. Binghamton: State University of New York Press.

Kleinman, Arthur. 1980. *Patients and Healers in the Context of Culture*. Los Angeles: UCLA Press.

Knipschild, P., J. Kleinen, and G. T. Riet. 1990. "Belief in the efficacy og alternative medicine among general practitioners in the Netherlands," *Social Science and Medicine*, 31:625–626.

Kronenfeld, J. J., and C. Wasner. 1982. "The use of unorthodox therapies and marginal practitioners," *Social Science and Medicine* 16:1119–1125.

Lepowsky, M. 1990. "Sorcery and penicillin: Treating illness on a Papua New Guinea island," *Social Science and Medicine* 30, 10:1049–1063.

Lim Tan, M. 1989. "Traditional or transitional medical systems? Pharmacotherapy as a case for analysis," *Social Science and Medicine* 29, 3:301–307.

Lissak, Moshe, and Dan Hurowitz. 1989. *Trouble in Utopia*. Albany: State University of New York Press.

Lock, Margaret. 1990. "Rationalization of Japanese herbal medication: The hegemony of orchestrated pluralism," *Human Organization* 49, 1:41–47.

Lock, Margaret, and Deborah Gordon (eds.).1988. *Biomedicine Examined*. Amsterdam: Kluwer Academic Publishers.

References

Lowenberg, J., and F. Davis.1994, "Beyond medicalisation-demedicalisation: The case of holistic health," *Sociology of Health and Illness* 16; 5:579–599.

Lupton, D. 1994. *Medicine as Culture.* London: Sage.

———. 1995. *The Imperative of Health.* London: Sage.

———. 1997. "Consumerism, reflexivity and the medical encounter," *Social Science and Medicine* 45, 3:373–381

Lyotard, J. F. 1987. " The post-modern condition." In K. Baynes, J. Bohman, and T. McCarty (eds.), *After Philosophy—End or Transformation?* Cambridge: MIT Press, 73–94.

McCannell, Dean. 1976. *The Tourist: A New Theory for the Leisure Class.* New York: Schoken.

McElroy, Ann, and Patricia Townsend. 1989. *Medical Anthropology in Ecological Perspective.* Boulder: Westview Press.

McGregor, Catherine, and Edmund Peay. 1996. "The choice of alternative therapy for health care: Testing some propositions," *Social Science and Medicine* 43, 9:1317–1327.

McGuire, Meredith. 1988. *Ritual Healing in Suburban America.* New Brunswick, NJ: Rutgers University Press.

McQueen, D. 1985. "China's impact on America's medicine in the seventies: A limited and preliminary enquiry," *Social Science and Medicine* 21, 8:931–936.

Maines, David. 1993. "Narrative's moment and sociology's phenomena: Toward a narrative sociology," *The Sociological Quarterly* 34, 1:17–38.

Martin, Emily. 1990. "The end of the body?," *American Ethnologist* February: 121–140.

Menges, L. J. 1994. "Regular and alternative medicine: the state of affairs in the Netherlands," *Social Science and Medicine* 39:871–873.

Miller, J. 1990. "Use of traditional Korean health care by Korean immigrants to the U.S.," *Society and Social Research* 75, 1:38–34.

Mills, S. Y. 2001. "Regulation in complementary and alternative medicine," *British Medical Journal* 322:158–160.

Mitchell, W. J. T. 1981. *On Narrative.* Chicago: University of Chicago Press.

Navarro, V. 1986. *Crisis, Health and Medicine: A Social Critique.* London: Tavistock.

New, P. K. 1977. "Traditional and modern health care: An appraisal of complementarity," *International Social Science Journal* 29, 3:483–496.

Novelli, W. 1990. "Controversies in the advertising of health-related products." In C. Atkin and L. Wallack (eds.), *Mass Communication and Public Health*. London: Sage.

Nudelman, A. 1993. "The importance of traditional healing for Ethiopian immigrants in Israel," *Collegium Anthropologicum* 17, 2:233–239.

Palgi, P. 1978. "Persistent traditional Yemenite ways of dealing with stress in Israel," *Mental Health and Society* 5:113–140.

Parsons, Talcot. 1966. *Societies, Evolutionary and Comparative Perspectives*. Englewood Cliffs, NJ: Prentice-Hall.

Perharic L., D. Shaw, and V. Murray. 1993. "Toxic effects of herbal medicines and food supplements," *The Lancet* 342, July 17:180–181.

Perkin, M. R., R. M. Pearcy, and J. S. Fraser. 1994. "A comparison of the attitudes shown by general practitioners, hospital doctors and medical students towards alternative medicine," *Journal of the Royal Society of Medicine* 87:525–527.

Pert, C. 1999. *Molecules of Emotion: The Science behind Mind-Body Medicine*. New York: Simon & Schuster.

Robertson, Roland. 1992. *Globalization: Social Theory and Global Culture*. London: Sage.

Ronen, M. 1988. "Alternative medicine as a functional alternative to western medicine," *Megamot* 33:252–265 (in Hebrew).

Said, Edward. 1978. *Orientalism*. New York: Pantheon

———. 1993, *Culture and Imperialism*. London: Vintage.

Saks, M. 1994. "The alternatives to medicine." In Gabe J., D. Kelleher, and G. Williams (eds.), *Challenging Medicine*. London: Routledge.

Schachter, L., M. Weingarten, and E. Kahan. 1993. "Attitudes of family physicians to non-conventional therapies," *Archives of Family Medicine* 2:1268–1270.

Schneirov, M., and J. D. Gezcik. 2002. "Alternative health and the challenges of instututionalization," *Social Science and Medicine* 6, 2:201–220.

Sered, Susan. 1988. "The domestication of religion: The spiritual guardianship of elderly oriental Jewish women," *Man* 23:506–521.

Sharma, Ursula. 1992. *Complementary Medicine Today—Practitioners and Patients* (rev. ed.). London: Routledge.

Shilling, Chris. 1993. *The Body and Social Theory*. London: Sage.

Shuval, J. T. 1980. "Professional socialization." In *Entering Medicine: A Seven Year Study of Medical Education in Israel*. New York: Pergamon, pp. 6–20.

References

Shuval, Judith, and Ofra Anson. 2000. *Social Structure and Health in Israel.* Jerusalem: The Hebrew University, Magnes Press.

Shvarts, Shifra. 2000. *Kupat Holim, Histadrut and the Government: The Formative Years of the Health System in Israel, 1947–1960.* Sede Boker: Ben-Gurion University of the Negev Press.

Signorelli, N. 1990. "Television and health: Images and impact." In C. Atkin and L. Wallack (eds.), *Mass Communication and Public Health.* London: Sage.

Sirois, F. M., and M. L. Gick. 2002. "An investigation of health beliefs and motivations of complementary medical clients," *Social Science and Medicine* 55:1025–1037.

Strauss, Anselm. 1987. *Qualitative Analysis for Social Scientists.* New York: Cambridge University Press.

Synott, A. 1992. "Tomb, temple, machine and self: the social construction of the body," *British Journal of Sociology* 43, 1:79–110.

———. 1993. *The Body Social: Symbolism, Self and Society.* London: Routledge.

Tobin, Joseph. 1992. "Introduction: Domesticating the West." In *Re-Made in Japan.* New Haven: Yale University Press, pp. 1–41.

Turner, Bryan. 1992. *Regulating Bodies: Essays in Medical Sociology.* London: Routledge.

———. 1994. *Orientalism, Postmodernism and Globalism.* London: Routledge.

———. 1995. *Medical Power and Social Knowledge.* London: Sage.

———. 1996. *The Body and Society.* London: Sage.

Unschuld, Peter. 1987. "Traditional Chinese medicine: Some historical and epistemological reflections," *Social Science and Medicine* 24, 12:1023–1029.

Urry, John. 1991. *The Tourist Gaze.* London: Sage.

Van Hemel, P. 2001. "A way out of the maze: Federal pre-emption of state licensing and regulation of complementary and alternative medicine practitioners," *American Journal of Law and Medicine* 27, 2–3:329–341.

Waitzkin, H. 1991. *The Politics of Medical Encounters.* New Haven: Yale University Press.

Wallerstein, Immanuel. 1974. *The Modern World System.* New York: Academic Press.

———. 1990. "Culture as the ideological battleground of the modern world-systems," *Theory, Culture and Society* 7, (2–3):31–55.

White, A. R., K. L. Resch, and E. Ernst. 1997. "Complementary medicine: Use and attitudes among GPs," *Family Practitioner* 14:302–306.

Williams, Simon. 1997."Modern medicine and the 'uncertain body': From corporeality to hyperreality?," *Social Science and Medicine* 45, 7:1041–1049.

Williams, S. J., and M. Calnan. 1996. "The limits of medicalization? Modern medicine and the lay populace in late modernity," in *Social Science and Medicine* 42, 12:1609–1620.

Wilson, Rob, and Wimal Dissanayake (eds.). 1996. *Global/Local: Cultural Production and the Transnational Imagery*. Durham: Duke University Press.

Zerubavel, Yael. 1996. *Recovered Roots*. Albany: State University of New York Press.

Index

acculturation, 10, 11, 17, 19, 20, 21, 22, 23, 26, 99, 108
affiliations
  academic, 98
  professional, 35, 39, 40
alternative medicine, 1, 2 (see non-conventional medicine)
antibiotics, 59, 85, 86, 93, 96
assimilation, 19, 20, 21, 22, 23
authenticity, 17, 18, 24, 86, 90, 114, 118

Baer, Hans, 2, 15, 19, 23, 25, 99, 108, 121, 126
Baer, Hans, Merrill Singer and Ida Susser, 5
Bauman, Zygmunt, 23, 130, 131
Bilu, Yoram, 11
biomedicine (conventional medicine), 1, 2
  and technology, 24
  authority of, 80, 90–95, 110, 115, 124
  criticism of, 86–90
  criticism of NCM, 92, 93
  culture of, 3, 20
  dissatisfaction with, 9, 12, 13, 14
  disappointment with, 127–128
  discourse of, 4
  dissemination of, 79
  globalization of, 5, 6, 23
  hegemony of, 10, 12, 13, 27, 33, 43, 49, 51, 55, 56, 60
  as meta-narrative, 130
  satisfaction with, 11
  socialization to, 3, 4, 97
  and technology, 24
body, the, 13, 24, 131, 134
  and holism, 133
  as energy, 104
  boundaries of, 133
  construction of, 102
  control of, 132
  dematerializing, 133
  objectification of, 91, 132
  patients' perception of, 74t
  power of healing, 102

Cant, Sarah and Ursula Sharma, 14, 15, 99, 100, 108, 126
charlatans, 29, 30, 31, 33, 94
China, 114, 121
Chinese medicine, 17, 18, 19, 101, 104
clinics (for non-conventional medicine)
  affiliations, 35, 39, 40
  bureaucracy, 34, 43, 45
  décor at, 40, 41
  domestication of, 34, 39
  dress code, 48
  public relations, 42
  sorting of patients, 44
  treatments available, 35, 44, 137–139
colleges (for non-conventional medicine)
  affiliations, 98
  décor, 101
  domestication, 100, 109, 115
  socialization, 99, 110
  staff, 110–111
  curriculum, 106–108
colonialism and bio-medicine, 5
Comaroff, Jean, 5
complementary medicine (see non-conventional medicine), 1, 2
consumerism, 13, 14, 117, 125, 129, 131
conventional medicine (see bio-medicine)
co-operation (bio-medicine and NCM), 15, 105, 109

Index

culture
  adaptation, 14, 16
  translation, 15, 35, 80
  counter-culture, 16, 21
curriculum, 106–108, 110

demedicalizationm, 13, 133
Deus ex Machina, 90
dissatisfaction,
  with CM, 9, 12–14, 127–128
  with NCM, 66
doctors (MDs) and NCM
  attitudes to, 5, 128
  practice of, 80, 85, 86, 95
  promotion of, 80
  referral of patients, 128
Doctors' Order (Israel), 28
doctor-patient relationship, 4, 18, 44, 46, 50, 53, 54, 120
domestication, 2, 5, 6, 9, 15, 16, 17, 19, 23, 24, 35, 82, 91, 100, 109, 113, 117, 118, 126, 127
Douglas, Mary, 13, 125

Eilon Commission, 28–32, 117
emotional problems, 94
empowerment (of patients), 87, 120
energy, 17, 89, 133, 134
epistemes (Foucault), 118

Featherstone, Mike, 5
Flexner Report, 97
Foucault, Michel, 3
fusion, 18, 91, 118
  biomedicine and NCM, 102, 106–107
  diagnosis and treatment, 107, 119, 120

Giddens, Anthony, 81, 130, 131
globalization, 3, 5, 6, 23
Good Byron, 3, 4, 97
grand narratives, 3, 130

Hannerz, Ulf, 5, 23, 24, 80, 131
healing, 89
hegemony,
  of bio-medicine, 10, 12, 13, 27, 33, 43, 49, 51, 56, 60
Hippocrates, 87, 90, 118, 123

holism, 4, 18, 24, 55, 60, 82, 91, 123, 128, 133
Homeopathy, 56, 57
  construction of symptoms, 58
  consultation, 56, 120
  professionalization, 100
  scientific paradigm, 100
  theory, 85, 99
hybridity, 5, 6, 18, 19, 23, 83, 84, 100, 106, 114–115, 117, 122

immigrants, 10, 11, 19, 21, 22, 25, 26
integration of modalities, 5, 16, 100, 123

Judaism in NCM, 27, 113

Kleinman, Arthur, 17, 64, 80

lifestyle, 65, 112, 113, 114, 123
Lock, Margaret, 126
Lupton, Deborah, 13, 120, 127

magic, 60–61
media
  dialogue between CM and NCM, 59, 82–83
  dissemination of NCM, 61, 82, 86
  NCM popularity in, 79
  NCM publicity in, 79
  support for NCM, 82
  as therapeutic community, 81, 83
medicalization, 87, 121, 129, 134
Medical Association of Israel (HARI), 32, 33, 79, 117, 129
medical gaze, 3, 24, 85, 90, 104
medications, 94
  self-medication, 93–94
medicine (see bio-medicine, non-conventional medicine)
melting-pot ideology and NCM, 25–27
mind-body connection, 55, 82, 88, 105, 128
modernization, 10–13, 124

narrative formulae, 83, 84
nutrition, 87
  mental well-being, 88
  physical well-being, 88

Index

non-conventional medicine, 1, 2
  co-operation with bio-medicine, 42, 86, 89, 90, 91, 95, 96
  as counter culture, 13
  cultural aspects of use, 65, 72, 76
  cultural mediation of, 15
  de-differentiation in Israel, 25–27
  dual use with CM, 67, 76, 125, 131
  discourse, 55
  disappointment with, 66
  incidence of use, 28, 63
  informal supervision of, 33, 34, 36
  legal status in Israel, 27, 98–99
  legitimation of, 96
  licensing, 15, 29
  lifestyle, 65
  as magic, 60
  efficacy, 93, 95
  professional titles, 110–111
  professional vocabulary, 108–110
  professionalization of, 21, 98, 99, 108, 119
  public relations, 43
  reasons for use, 64, 75
  and scientific authority, 103
  socialization of students, 111
  supervision of practice, 30, 32
  theories of recourse to, 6–9, 10–16, 64, 75

Orientalismm 18, 23, 103

paradoxes,
  empowerment and objectification, 24, 87, 90, 134
  inefficacy and harm, 93, 95
paternalism, 94–95, 125
patients of NCM
  abuse by NCM practitioners, 94
  attitudes to bio-medicine, 68, 69
  attitudes to NCM, 73t
  compliance with NCM, 44, 46, 50, 54, 56, 59
  as consumers, 74–75
  cultural profile, 125
  demographic characteristics, 68–69t
  health problems, 69
  quantitative studies of, 65
  satisfaction with MD, 70, 71t
  lifestyle, 76

placebo, 59, 60, 94, 95
pluralism, 9, 14, 15
postmodernity, 2, 13, 24, 81, 130, 134–135
practitioners of NCM, 21
  and co-operation with MDs, 47, 49, 50
professionalization of NCM, 21, 98, 99, 108, 119
  professional titles, 110–111
  professional vocabulary, 108–110
psycho-neuro-immunology, 128
psychosomatic complaints, 53, 55, 132

Said, Edward, 18, 23, 103
Sharma, Ursula, 64
socialization of students
  to NCM, 109, 111
  to bio-medicine, 3, 4, 97, 98
sociological theory and NCM, 6–9, 10–16, 64, 75
State Ombudsman's report (Israel), 32
supervision of NCM
  informal regulation, 33, 34, 36
  legal status in Israel, 27, 98–99
  legitimation of, 96
  licensing, 15, 29
  of practice, 30, 32
symptoms, construction of
  in bio-medicine, 5, 57
  in NCM, 102, 103, 123

terminology, 1–2
traditional medicine, 9, 10, 11, 22, 26, 126
treatments (description of),
  chiropractic, 137
  herbs, 138
  homeopathy, 138
  Meyer method, 138
  Paula technique, 138
  natural holistic medicine, 139–140
  nutrition, 139
  reflexology, 139
Turner, Brian, 23, 24, 80, 131

Unschuld, Paul, 17

Waitzkin, Howard, 5